Hoarders

Family and Friends Guide to Dealing With Their Hoarder {Large Print}

By Hoarder Susan L. Harrington

Thank you to my friend and editor, "Dallas Ann" Blackbourn for editing this book.

After multiple edits, if you find a typo, please Email: storiesforpublication@yahoo.com. Thank you!

If you have found tips to help your loved one or friend, who just happens to be a hoarder, please go to amazon.com or Kindle and write a 5-star review so that others can be helped by this book.

Hoarders

Family and Friends Guide to Dealing With Their Hoarder

Introduction

I am a hoarder. Been that way for decades. Not bad enough to get on television, but bad enough to cause friction in relationships—and embarrassment if I don't get "stuff" shoved into my bedroom fast enough when there's a knock at the door. My bedroom? It's off limits all of the time.

My 92-year old Mother is a hoarder. My Dad and his brother were both hoarders, too.

I'm assuming that you are a family member, former family member, or a friend of a hoarder.

As a hoarder, I am so grateful that you care enough to read this book. It is my intent that by the end of the book, you will have a better understanding of hoarders so that you can help your hoarder and not drive them away.

In this book I will share about hoarding and suggestions on ways to help your hoarder so they don't go into a hoarding tailspin.

> **Please do not jump to the 2nd or 3rd part of the book. If you do not understand the mind of your hoarder, you might say or do the wrong thing which might alienate your hoarder worse—and they go on a hoarding buying spree.**

A lot of tips and techniques are repeated over and over again. It's important for you to fully grasp and implement these tips and techniques so that you will be less frustrated and your loved one will reduce their clutter.

This book is divided up into three distinct sections:

Part I: Discusses what hoarding is, the difference between hoarding and collecting, medical reasons for hoarding, a hoarding quiz, types of hoarding, and the cause of hoarding.

Part II: ***Please read Part I before reading either Part II or Part III or you will miss some important information when dealing with your hoarder loved one.*** Part II discusses some of the instances when you must step in as well as how to help your hoarder downsize specific items.

Part III: To get the most out of this book and to help your hoarder in the fastest way possible, you should read Part I first followed by Part II and then read Part III which discusses how to help your hoarder by working in zones.

Disclaimer: I am not a medical professional or a counselor. I am just a researcher who happens to be a hoarder. By reading this book you accept and understand that neither the author, publisher, or printer is responsible, in any way, for any information in this book nor any information omitted from this book. It is the sole responsibility of the reader to seek any and all professional physical, mental, and/or spiritual help that their loved one, who is a hoarder, might need. The author is sharing her experiences as a hoarder and provides suggestions, only, on what you might do to help your hoarder reduce their clutter.

Table of Contents

Part I

Hoarding: What is it?

Hoarding is the excessive collecting of alive items such as animals or non-alive items which could be anything else. Some of the most frequent items that hoarder's hang onto are books, clothing, magazines, newspapers, and paperwork.

I am a hoarder of all of the above items with clothing being the least hoarded item. Periodically I am able to go through my clothes to downsize them.

> Even some non hoarders will save several sizes of jeans and slacks hoping that "someday" that they will get back in them.

The Difference Between Hoarding and Collecting

It's possible to be both a hoarder and a collector, but I'm just going to explain a simplified distinction between the two.

A collector generally collects one or two types of items such as stamps, coins, dolls, trains, salt and pepper shakers, etc. Generally, their collections are organized and don't overtake the entire house.

If something traumatic happens in a collector's life, their collecting can shift into hoarding. What happens, then, is their collections become disorganized, and can randomly spill out into the rest of their home, garage, and/or yard. Their items appear to give them more emotional pleasure than people and they appear to have an emotional overreaction to their collected items.

Hoarding is having an emotional attachment to things. Usually clutter just overtakes their home with little to no organization to their possessions.

Medical Reasons for Hoarding

Yes, there are medical reasons which might cause your loved one to hoard. You need to rule out these medical conditions, first, before you deal with the hoarding. It's possible, that if your loved one is hoarding, due to a medical reason, and the medical reason is taken care of, your loved one may, on their own, deal with their hoarding.

Dementia: There are many causes of reversible dementia such as dehydration, dental problems, medication interactions, urinary tract infections, plus many more. Especially if your loved one is a senior, I strongly encourage you to purchase the amazing, eye-opening book, by speaker/author Susan L. Harrington, titled: "Broken Brain: Caretakers Guide to Alzheimer's and Other Dementias" which is available on amazon.com and Kindle. (You can also review this book, and many other types of books, at: www.storiesforpublication.com.)

If your hoarder has a reversible dementia, once the medical condition is fixed, then their minds will revert back to normal and they may clean up their hoarding piles on their own.

If their doctor has ruled out dehydration, dental problems, medicine interactions, urinary tract infections, and other medical conditions that cause dementia, which might have a side effect of confusion, then they probably don't have reversible dementia. (Confusion can cause a person to forget that they purchased something so they buy more of the same item.)

<u>Depression</u>: Another medical condition in which the end result could be what appears to be hoarding is depression. If a person is depressed, then it's just too much effort for them to put items away and clutter accumulates making the person appear to be a hoarder. Technically, a hoarder has emotional attachments to items which you might think of as junk. If a person has a household full of clutter, because they are depressed and it's just too much effort to keep their home clean, and they do not have an extreme emotional attachment to the clutter, then they are not a hoarder. In this case, once the depression is helped, then they should clean up their clutter.

You aren't going to like what I'm about to say. Speaking as a hoarder, you—being our loved ones and our so-called friends can depress us. You think you are helping us, but when you threaten us about our hoarding, or nag us about our hoarding, or are judgmental about our hoarding, it's extremely painful being around you. You don't get it that when you treat us like that, you are crushing us, and that to soothe us your actions might even send us into a hoarding-buying frenzy. We might even begin to wonder if you even love us or if you just get a kick out of bullying us. If this shocks you, then you may be just the person to shift your actions and reactions to your loved one, who just happens to be a hoarder. You might actually be the person who can lovingly help your hoarder regain their life back! You don't have to understand your hoarder to help them. In fact you may never understand hoarding. That's okay. I don't understand how a car runs, but I still drive my car.

Other conditions that _may_ also have hoarding as a side effect are people who have been diagnosed with schizophrenia, Tourette's syndrome, or obsessive-compulsive disorder (OCD). It's important for you to not assume that your loved one also has one of these other conditions. The only way to know for sure if they also have these conditions is for them to get tested. Once these conditions are treated, the person may reduce their hoarding on their own.

<u>I'm not telling you other conditions, so you can tease your loved one further about these, too</u>. I'm telling you so that, if you really love your loved one, that you can help, not hurt further. So that you can be supportive, not harassing. If you respond back that you are just teasing, stop! Your teasing is cruel and hurtful and painful. You are driving your loved one away. They wonder if you really even love them. What they feel by your words, actions, and even your tone of voice, is that you are a bully. That you are judgmental. That you don't really love them. If you are willing—and want to change so that they know that you do love them, then read this book. It just may transform your life and the life of your loved one!

Hoarding Quiz

This is a simple questionnaire to see if your loved one may be a hoarder. The questionnaire is not intended to shame them; it's to give you a starting point in dealing with hoarding. This is an unscientific quiz. <u>Remember, first you need to ensure that your loved one doesn't have a medical reason for hoarding</u>.

1. Is your loved one always losing things in their clutter? (You have to ensure that they do not have dementia. Early onset dementia can occur in adults under the age of 60.)

2. Does your loved one get defensive if you offer to help them clean their home? (It might not be that they don't want your help; it could be that by your so-called teasing, threatening, nagging, and overall disrespect of them and their possessions, that what you consider help, is just the opposite to your loved one.)

3. Does your loved one have difficulty keeping their car, kitchen table, bedroom, or other area clear of clutter? (We almost

<u>all</u> have problems with some form of clutter. It's when the clutter, which may be considered junk to others, has an over-emotional attachment to us.)

4. If you open your loved one's refrigerator, is there moldy or dried up food inside or on the counter? (This is not true with all hoarders and may be, instead, a sign of depression or dementia.)

5. Does your loved one have difficulty throwing out junk mail, magazines, or other paper? (It's the emotional attachment to items that is one of the biggest indicators that your loved one may be a hoarder.)

If you answered yes to at least two questions, and you have ruled out medical reasons for your loved one's clutter, your loved one <u>may be</u> a hoarder. This information is not shared with you so that you may use it against your loved one. Instead, it is a non-scientific possible indicator so that, hopefully, you can step up to the plate and say that you really, really, want to help your loved one, who is a hoarder.

I am so happy that you are reading this book! Because, if <u>you read and apply</u> what I'm about to share with you, you <u>may</u> see a transformation so shocking, that you may think of it as a miracle! Realize that your loved one may want help, but only if it is lovingly done and that you respect them and their possessions.

Types of Hoarding

The different experts list several different types of hoarding disorders. I will list some of the main types of hoarding. You just need to realize that some professionals might call specific types of hoarding by a different name. All you care about is that you can identify what your loved one's preference is for hoarding.

In parts two and three of this book, I will break these large categories of hoarding down to more manageable hoarding preferences and share with you some ideas which have worked for me as well as suggestions on how you can help and not hurt your loved one who just happens to be a hoarder.

I can confirm what I'm about to share with you. When I'm going to a garage sale or a church sale, I get so excited with the anticipation of possibly finding a bargain that I have to restrain myself from running to the sale. It's been researched that endorphins are released which give us a high; a feeling of euphoria. Once we purchase the item, or order the item, the high can quickly dissipate. In fact, by the time we drive in the driveway with our new possessions, the high might be totally gone. That's why you might see items still with the tags on or boxes and packages unopened in a hoarder's home. The high is gone and they have lost interest in the item.

<u>Animal Hoarding</u>: We love our animals. Just in the United States, alone, over 1/3 of us own a dog or a cat. It becomes hoarding when somebody collects dozens—or even hundreds of animals. The key here is that your loved one cannot adequately take care of all of their animals. The animals might be underfed, diseased, and/or the house may have feces on the floor and on other surfaces. (If a person has dementia, they lose concept of time and they think they fed/walked/cleaned up after their pets when they haven't. That's why it's important to have your loved one checked out by medical personnel.)

<u>Collection Hoarding</u>: The hoarder may have started out just collecting one or two things and then something happens in your loved one's life. The collection outgrows the space and spills out into the rest of the house, garage, and/or yard or the collector gets bored with one collection and moves to another collection and they run out of room. The distinction is that the collection, which has overtaken the house has disrupted normal living, which is one of the symptoms of hoarding.

<u>Food Hoarding</u>: This may also be called larder hoarding. It's wise to have excess non-perishable food and water on hand in case of a natural disaster. People who call themselves "Preppers" stockpile food. They are not necessarily considered food hoarders. Food hoarders stockpile food that they couldn't possibly eat before the expiration dates on the food. Food may be piled all over the house with no organization to it. Food inside of their refrigerator may be spoiled and food in their freezer may have freezer burn.

Before you just assume that your loved one is a food hoarder, think about it first. If you, personally, do not keep spare food items on hand, you might falsely judge others who do. Not everybody who purchases food on sale and has multiple cans or boxes of the same food item is a food hoarder.

Even though I am a hoarder, I do not consider myself a food hoarder. I have a small pantry filled with food and in the spare room, there is one shelving unit with food on each shelf. The food is organized and the expiration dates are marked on each items. The cans and boxes that expire the soonest are closest to the edge of the shelf. I consider it wiser to purchase food on sale rather paying full price for it. So even though I may purchase a case of an item on sale, I try to purchase what will be eaten prior to the expiration date. I don't always succeed, but I try. Likewise, in the refrigerator and freezer I may occasionally misjudge and some food may wilt, however, I don't have a compulsion to keep spoiled food. I don't get anxious if say cans of corn get down to a certain number; I just make note to purchase more cans of corn the next time they are on sale.

Recycling Hoarding: Another name for recycling hoarders is "non-wasters". Recycling is a good thing which we should all do. With recycling hoarders their house and often their yard is littered with one or more types of items that could be recycled such as plastic, glass, paper, copper, steel, and other items that can be recycled. Someday they plan to take the items to turn it into cash. The problem is that their someday never comes and the recyclable items never get off of the property. Their intent is good; their follow through is almost nonexistent. With hoarders, they see the items that are taking over their home and yard;

however, they don't understand that their excessive clutter is a trip hazard, a fire hazard, and could be a health hazard.

<u>Researcher Hoarding</u>: Those of us who love to read and research may have piles of books magazines, newspapers, and even encyclopedias. I am an author, researcher, and love to read.   I have probably have over a thousand books, and boxes of newspapers and magazines.   Thankfully, I don't have encyclopedias—except for a medical encyclopedia. In the next section, I will share what works for me to downsize my researcher hoarding.

<u>Shopping Hoarding</u>: Sometimes a shopping hoarder is also called a shopper hoarder. They might joke that they are a shopaholic. A shopping hoarder save everything they purchase even when what they buy they don't have any use for it.   They may love the shopping network shows and their house and garage may be stacked with unopened boxes that they purchased. Basically this includes the over purchasing everything from food to collectibles to clothing to anything on the shopping networks. Note: a person can be a shopping hoarder and not even watch the shopping networks. Shopping becomes hoarding when it effects their daily living and they have an emotional attachment to the items they hoard. Not always, but due to their hoarding, a shopping hoarder can be in debt. Their shopping hoarding can cause trip hazards, health and hygiene hazards, fire hazards as well as other issues.

Two other categories which the experts might list are what's called over-sentimental hoarders and typical hoarders. Personally, I'm not too thrilled with these two categories. To a hoarder, they can be considered over-sentimental over everything. If you try to throw away a piece of scratch paper of a paper hoarder, they are going to feel disrespected and violated. To me, being over-sentimental is a symptom and not a category.

Also, I don't consider the phrase typical hoarders to be an overall category. To me, it just means that some of the most common things that hoarders may hoard are: animals, clothing, paper, magazines, newspapers, and collections gone awry.

The only reason I list them, here, is for you to know what some of the experts say.

The Cause of Hoarding

I could not find any conclusive evidence that one specific thing causes hoarding; meaning there could be and there is a good indication that there is more than one reason why loved ones become hoarders. Three areas of research are: activity in the brain, genetics, and/or trauma in the hoarder's life.

<u>Activity in the brain</u>: Being a hoarder and a researcher, I took notice when I read about a controlled research study by a team lead by a man called Tolin. What was fascinating about their research was the fact that they used what's called functional MRIs or fMRIs. These special MRIs allowed them to immediately tract and record brain activity when the subjects were put through hoarding stressful conditions as well as situations that were not stressful for hoarders. They also had people who were not hoarders go through the same testing. This experiment caused more "anxiety, indecisiveness and sadness" among hoarders. He also said that they avoid doing anything about their clutter because it is too "painful".

While you think that hoarders should just have self-control and clean up their clutter, I'm practically jumping up and down pumping my arm saying "Yes!" Remember Tolin had immediate brain-activity images from the fMRIs.

> The fMRIs are scientific proof that there is a physical reason (brain activity) why we hoard. It's validating to have scientific proof that hoarders aren't lazy.

In hoarder's brains, part of their brain was over stimulated and part of their brain was under stimulated. The part of their brain that was over stimulated was hoarder's reactions to getting rid of the stuff that they hoard. On the other hand, the part of their brain that was under stimulated was their lack of seeing all of their clutter and mess as a problem.

For those of you more technical readers, the over stimulation occurred in two distinct parts of the brain; the anterior cingulate cortex and the left insular cortex. He further concluded that hoarders who had been diagnosed with either depression and/or OCD, which is obsessive-compulsive disorder, had no relevance to the research study. In simplified terms, it means that if a person is depressed or they also have OCD, which is common in some hoarders, depression and OCD didn't cause the over- and under-stimulation in parts of their brain. Or put another way, depression and OCD did not alter the brain activity when they looked at activities that normally would either make a hoarder anxious or not anxious.

He concluded that those two parts of the brains directly affect how the brain processes information about clutter. When the brain is over stimulated, like when you want to take away our possessions (clutter), we get overly anxious.   When the hoarder looks at their clutter, that part of the brain which processes the information is under stimulated, which means that although they see the clutter, it doesn't bother them. To put it into perspective, look at a chair. Your brain registers that it is a chair, with no other reaction, and then your attention moves to something else. That's how our brain relates to clutter. We see the clutter, but because it doesn't register in our brain that it's a bad thing which could jeopardize our safety and quality of life, we just ignore our clutter.   Because of the way the study was conducted; using control subjects (people who weren't hoarders) and because they used fMRIs, which immediately recorded brain activity, as a hoarder, this makes sense to me as being a valid reason why we hoard.

<u>Genetics</u>: There's research that believes that up to 50% of hoarding comes from a genetic influence. Some of the research is targeting chromosome 14 for hoarding. The research was not conclusive; meaning that at this time the researchers are not 100% positive that something to do with chromosome 14 indicates hoarding. Whether or not researchers prove for sure that chromosome 14 is an indicator for hoarding, anybody who has studied family psychology knows that children tend to mimic those adults in our life. We've probably all seen a little boy try to imitate the way his father walks or sits. Since most of the hoarding tends to start in the impressionable teenage years, the teenager might just be mimicking the adult's hoarding behavior. Like I said, both of my parents were hoarders as well as my uncle on my father's side. Later I will share information that might help you to help your hoarder reduce some of their clutter.

<u>Trauma</u>: Everybody has things that happen to them; that is part of life. When the past trauma affects how we live our current life, it's labeled post traumatic syndrome. For example, a child might have lived with neglect and abuse. If they were often hungry, as a child, they might have this fear of being hungry so they hoard food.

Or, if they grew up in poverty, they might hoard things to prove to themselves that they aren't that poor neglected child anymore.   If a child experienced abuse in their childhood, they had no control over those experiences, and might seek comfort—and validation in things. Now, as an adult, hoarding gives them temporary pleasure; stuff brings comfort to them; even if it's for a few moments.

There is mounting evidence that as adults if we have a traumatic experience, one way that we might cope with it is to start hoarding. Even though most of the hoarding starts when we are a teenager, a traumatic event when we are an adult can trigger something in our brain and we start hoarding.   Some events, which might trigger the hoarding response or reaction is: abuse or attacks, divorce, death of someone who is close to them, having their house burn down, a natural disaster, or other events that are traumatic to that individual. What you must understand is that when a person has a traumatic event, it doesn't necessarily mean that they will become a hoarder. However, if you are a loved one of an adult who has recently gone through a traumatic event and you start noticing more clutter in their home, they might be starting to turn to hoarding to provide comfort to themselves.

Risk Factors

Similar to most types of dementia[1], even though a family member has dementia, or is a hoarder, it doesn't mean that a person will 100% get dementia or become a hoarder.

Some of the most common risk factors are:

Age. Generally hoarding starts when a person is a teenager and gets worse as a person ages. That's one reason why hoarding is more prevalent in older adults than their younger counterparts.

If you think that just because a loved one is now living in assisted living or a care center (nursing home), don't wrongly assume that they won't hoard anymore. Not true. A few years ago we helped a friend move her mother to a closer assisted living facility. As we were packing her up, we found lots of candy, packaged cookies and crackers, and fruit squirreled away hidden in different places. Many pieces of fruit were found, especially bananas, which were in various stages of rot. One banana had been there so long that it was completely dried out with its shriveled up black outer skin the only evidence that it had once been a banana.

<u>Family</u>. If a person lives with a hoarder, they have a higher risk factor of becoming a hoarder. This is a fact.

<u>Personality Traits</u>. Many hoarders either have problems making decisions or they are perfectionists. Many hoarders feel that if we get rid of something, we might need it later so we keep practically everything; many items that others feel are outdated, spoiled, or have no value. Many people are surprised when they hear that some hoarders are perfectionists. People wrongly assume that if that were true, then the hoarder would want everything orderly and not in a constant state of chaos.   If a hoarder is a perfectionist, they have such a fear of making the wrong decision, they make no decision at all and the clutter piles up in their home.

<u>Trauma</u>. If somebody has had extreme neglect and/or abuse, or if they were or felt abandoned or not loved in their past, they have an increased risk of becoming a hoarder. As an adult, a traumatic event can trigger them to become a hoarder.   Some of those events

could include being attacked or robbed, the death of somebody close to them, losing their job, divorce, a natural disaster, or their home burning down.

---

1   "Broken Brain: Caretakers Guide to Alzheimer's and Other Dementias" by Susan L. Harrington.

Pitfalls of Being a Hoarder

If you are a non-hoarder, you just don't get it. You don't understand why we hoard and why we just can't stop hoarding. You don't have to understand your hoarder to learn some tips to help your hoarder. I'm going to share just a few of the pitfalls of being a hoarder.

<u>Family strain and conflict</u>. Because family members don't understand the dynamics that the hoarders feel, they do the wrong thing and tell the hoarder to clean up their mess. They threaten their loved one. They are judgmental. And their help comes across as bullying—and unloving.

Suggestion: Right now, stop telling your hoarder what to do. Quit nagging them. Quit judging them. Quit trying to help them by your standards and not theirs. Today, right now, if you love your loved one, who just happens to be a hoarder, treat them with dignity and respect. Ask and not tell. After you read and absorb the information in this book, if you want to nag somebody, nag other family members and friends of your hoarder to read this book.

<u>Social Isolation</u>: Because family and friends nag and judge the hoarder, the loved one tends

to withdraw from social functions with family and friends.

Suggestion: Treat your hoarder with dignity and respect. Call them up just to say hi and don't mention their clutter and mess. If your loved one likes a certain restaurant, ask them if they would like to meet you there. Ask other family members to initiate contact with their loved one and to not mention, to their hoarder, their clutter and mess.

<u>Loneliness and shame</u>: I don't think family members and friends of hoarders understand how much their harping about the hoarder's mess hurts them and shames them. Other's negative actions and reactions towards them makes them feel more lonely and shamed.

Suggestion: A hoarder is much more than just a hoarder. It should just be one thing that defines them like they are a golfer or they have brown hair. Hoarding shouldn't be the only thing that defines them in your eyes. Treat your hoarder like a sister or brother, an uncle or an aunt, a daughter or a son, or a friend and not just a hoarder.

<u>Risk of falls</u>: Depending on how severe the hoarding is in their home, the risk of falls

increases. Stacks of clutter can shift and fall into the pathway and the loved one can trip and fall. Also, your loved one can be distracted or forget that they placed something in a certain place and then trip and fall.

Suggestion: Read this book cover-to-cover. Implement as many of the suggestions as you can. But you cannot rush your loved one. You have to work within their time tolerance, which is the amount of sorting or cleaning time before your loved one gets grumpy because their anxiety level is increasing. If you are visiting your loved one, and you see a trip hazard, ask if you can clear the path because you care about them and don't want them to fall and hurt themselves. Remember to not complain about the clutter.

<u>Risk of injury from falling items</u>: The higher the items are stacked, the risk increases that the items can shift and fall on your loved one. Depending on how heavy the falling item is, they may be hurt or even pinned underneath the item.

Suggestion: Renew contact with your loved one. If you talk to them a certain time each day or week and you cannot reach them, then you need to take immediate action to make sure that they haven't fallen in their home or had something fall on them.

<u>Health risks</u>: Depending on what items your loved one hoards, they may have spoiled food in the house that they are eating. If your loved one is an animal hoarder, and the animals are excreting inside of their home, there are additional health risks. Just the added dust may increase the risk of respiratory illnesses.

Suggestion: There are suggestions within this book on how to deal with food hoarding, animal hoarding, and reducing clutter in the life of your loved one in ways that they can handle—and that makes sense to them. If it doesn't make sense to your loved one, then they won't do it.

<u>Eviction risk</u>: If a loved one is a renter and people complain because either their apartment stinks from rotten food or animal wastes or because their yard is unsightly due to all of the clutter in their yard, it increases their risk of being evicted.

Suggestion: Don't shame your loved one by calling them a filthy pig. Be part of the solution and not the problem. Read the book and try to implement some of the many suggestions to help your loved one reduce their clutter and regain their dignity.

<u>Fines risks</u>: If your loved one's clutter spills out into their yard, they won't be able to mow their lawn according to city ordinances. Many cities and towns have ordnances about unsightly yards, which could include fines.

Suggestion: If you are worried about your loved one getting fined for their clutter, then you can offer to help them using the suggestions from this book. (Read this book <u>before</u> you offer to help your loved one.)

<u>Fire hazards</u>: If a loved one's home is full of flammable material, i.e. paper, newspapers, magazines, and other items, and especially if your loved one smokes, the fire risks increase significantly. Limited pathways within their home may make it more difficult for your loved one to escape if there is a fire. Doors may be blocked with piles or boxes of clutter. Because of the clutter, your loved one may not be able to change the batteries in their smoke alarms.

Suggestion: Do not nag them that they live in a fire trap. Instead offer to help in loving, nonjudgmental ways that are discussed in this book.

Part II

When you must step in

How to help your hoarder: specific items

When You Must Step In

I don't like this section and your loved one won't either. Be advised that if you step in, do so cautiously, because all hell might break loose. If your loved one was bullied or abused in their past, they might think you are just carrying on the abuse by stepping in—and literally stealing their animals or stuff that they have an emotional attachment to.

You're going to come across as demon possessed, a hypocrite, a bully, threatening, nagging, unfair, a thief, and/or other negative terms in the mind of your loved one.

Animal Hoarding: You are taking away animals that they love. Your loved one may never forgive you for the evil you are doing to them by stealing their pets that they love so much. You are treating them with disrespect. You are being a nag.

Having said that, however, if your loved one is an animal hoarder, and there are animal feces on the floor and other surfaces, the cat litter pan is always totally full of poop, and/or the animals look uncared for and hungry, then it's time to step in.

You might try to soften the blow, by asking them which is their favorite dog or cat—or whatever type of animal your loved one hoards.

When you steal their pets away from them, which is taking the pets away from them against their will, treat your loved one and all of the pets that you are taking from them, with dignity and respect. Don't complain about it when you are trying to cage the pets. Whatever you do, don't get the media involved so that your loved one is shamed, even more, on the evening news when they show pictures of animals being crated and being removed from their home.

Be advised, that if you steal their pets, then they will start collecting more pets as soon as they can. When they do, it has nothing to do with you; it's their hoarding instinct kicking in. Their pets do not bully them like you do. Their pets don't steal from them (by removing their pets) like you do. Their pets don't judge them like you do.

Neglect of Children: This is probably going to come to a total shock to you. It doesn't make sense to you; it's not logical. You think we are an unfit parent so you threaten us and eventually take away our children or other dependents—and we let you. You think that we love our junk more than our children. No--you are <u>TOTALLY</u> wrong!

You steal our children and you break our hearts. You rip out our hearts when you steal our children from us. We are devastated and you wrongly think that we love our junk more than we love our children. You are so wrong…

Please stop and reread the first two paragraphs of this section.   You disrespect us.   You threaten us. You bully us. You nag us. **No matter what you think, in our minds we are victims**.   We don't want you to steal our children.

> We let you take our children because we feel like we have no other options.

We don't trust you. We feel that since you have been bullying us, shaming us, and nagging us, even if we were to clean up our clutter that it wouldn't matter. In our minds you want to steal our children. In our minds you will find some other way to steal our children from us and nothing we do can change your minds. So, since we are victims, we do nothing. It's a terrible, terrible thing you do to us when you steal our children. You break our hearts. Most likely, to comfort us, we will hoard more.

> Things don't break our hearts like you have just done to us.

We may feel so much pain, afterwards, that our hoarding may actually get worse because the hoarding may temporarily ease our pain.

How To Help Your Hoarder

*****If you immediately jumped to this section, without reading the rest of the book, I strongly encourage you to take the time to go back and start from the beginning of the book.***** You might find that your hoarder has some other medical condition that once fixed, they reduce their clutter on their own.

Whether you are a man or a woman, what you've read might actually have made you cry when you realize that how you have been treating your loved one, to them, is far from in a loving behavior. You wrongly felt that what you did was showing love towards your loved one who is also a hoarder. Unfortunately, your hoarder might even wonder if you even do love them. That is exactly why I have written this book; to help you and your loved one deal with their hoarding in a way which will help them and empower them.

If you live with a hoarder, tread softly. If you've already been nagging them about their clutter, stop immediately! If you nag them, yet you leave dirty clothes on the floor or leave empty food wrappers around the house or in the car, your loved one thinks you are a bully and a hypocrite. They think that you have double standards and that you are trying to make them live according to what you consider is neat. (You said that you wanted to help your loved one. If you really do, you will not get defensive about what I'm trying to tell you; you will heed what I'm saying. This book is about your loved one—and trying to help them with their hoarding.)

If you tell your hoarder that you are coming to help them get rid of their junk, this one of the worse things you can say to them. Why? You are not asking; you are ordering them. You are disrespecting them by calling their possessions junk. When you talk to your loved one like that, their anxiety level skyrockets. In their mind, you are charging into their life, uninvited, and are going to steal their possessions. Yes, if you take their possessions, without their permission, you are technically stealing their stuff. It doesn't matter that in your mind that it is junk. To them it isn't.

Let's put it in perspective. Say you had an old Mustang that you were in the process of restoring. Right now it has rust on the outside, a broken taillight, and ripped seats. How would you feel if somebody came in and took your

Mustang you were restoring, without your permission, and took it to the scrapyard because it was, in their eyes, junk? You'd be pissed, wouldn't you? Well, to your loved one, even though you think their stuff is junk, to them it's not. You have to treat them and their stuff with respect.

What <u>not</u> to do:

1. Threaten them that if they don't clean up their mess, you will ________________.
(Stop talking to your loved one like this. You are disrespecting them by treating them like a child.)

2. Don't charge into their home, with garbage bags, and without their permission, fill up the garbage bags and haul off the junk. (Again, you are treating them like a child. You are disrespecting your loved one. Technically, you are stealing their stuff.)

3. Don't tell your loved one that you are coming over to help them to clean up their house. (You are bossing your loved one around. You are disrespecting them. Since they know that you are judging

them, negatively, their anxiety and stress level skyrockets and by the time you get to their house they will really be stressed out.)

4. When one family member takes your loved one to a doctor's appointment, and then other family members come in and clean their loved ones house to surprise them, it's not a good surprise. (How would you like it if somebody came into your home and threw out whatever they liked without asking your permission first? You wouldn't like it. Well, your loved one won't like it either.) Yes, you had good intentions, but this isn't the way to go about it. You are still disrespecting your loved one by throwing away their stuff without their permission.

Ways to work **with** your loved one. The key is working with your loved one. You love your loved one and you really do want to help them.

An important thing to remember is that we only have a certain length of time that we can work on the clutter before our stress level increases and we get grumpy. For me, my limit is around 40 minutes. Depending on how old your loved one is, their stress time tolerance level may only be 10-15 minutes. Honor that and at the end of their tolerance level stop and praise them for what <u>they</u> got accomplished. You are never are going to accomplish what you want to accomplish; that's not the point. The point is that you are spending time with your loved one, respecting them, and honoring their time tolerance level. In the meantime your relationship with your loved one should strengthen and slowly, their clutter should be reduced.

> No matter what your loved one hoards, if they agree to donate, recycle, shred it, or remove the item (throw it away), <u>always</u> take the items <u>every</u> time you leave or they might take it out of the boxes and hide the items.

As a hoarder, I'm going to share some ideas with you. I'm going to share some real-life stories with you too. Remember, everybody's temperament is different. Talk with your loved one to find out what works for them. The key is here is communication. You don't tell; you ask. You don't judge; you help—always with your loved one's permission.

To you, you see a house filled with junk. Stacks and stacks of junk. Remember, it's not about you—it's about your loved one. Bite your tongue. Don't criticize them or judge them. Don't mumble under your breath. If you do, your so-called helping them actually will do more hoarding damage and the increased anxiety level, by you disrespecting them by your comments and attitudes, may actually cause them to go on an additional hoarding frenzy after you leave.

Your loved one has a conscious or subconscious rating on what they hoard. Say your loved one hoards address labels, envelopes, books, magazines, and newspapers. What you think would mean the most to them, might not be the case. We are not dealing with logic here; we are dealing with the emotional attachment to certain items. The best thing to do is to ask your loved one, in a calm nonjudgmental voice, either which ones, listing the items, either mean the most or the least to them. To have the highest level of success and less relapse, leave the most emotional-based items for last and first work with your loved one on the items that have the least emotional attachment to them. <u>What you must get—and fully accept and understand, is</u>

that even though address labels may have the least emotional attachment to them, they still do mean something to them or they wouldn't be collected and hoarded.

I will list the types of clutter by alphabetical order. I'm also giving you some minor hoarding items, which might be easier for your hoarder to work with. For example, one of the hoarding items I'm listing are address label hoarding. In your mind you want to clean up the mess in the house, attic, garage, and/or yard. But, you need to realize that some hoarding items will be easier for your loved one to part with than others. For me, books are very important to me. If I was forced to start with books, it would be too painful to me to do and therefore more likely to backfire. But, if I started with something that has less emotional significance to me, then I would more likely be open to working on that item, first, and work up to the books. The thing is, that if I'm encouraged and not shamed and praised instead of shamed, then on my own I might feel stronger to work on downsizing my thousands of books on my own.

You don't have to read every word of this section; however, it will be easier—on you and your hoarder, if you start with individual items

<u>and work up to zones</u>. You will soon notice that I repeat concepts and suggestions. I do this on purpose because what I'm sharing with you, because I am a hoarder, is so important that you must get it.

> You want to start with a big zone, which is an area. No! If you do, you will get frustrated and your loved one will get so anxious, the sorting session will cease. Instead, you need to start with baby steps, which will build up your loved one's tolerance level. Trust me; I know because I am a hoarder.

<u>Address Label Hoarding</u>: My Mother is on all sorts of mailing lists and she receives hundreds of address labels. I recently opened up a cabinet and address labels went all over the place. She had literally thousands of address labels. I didn't judge her. I didn't yell at her. I picked up the address labels off of the floor and brought several inches of address labels over to the dining room table. I gently explained to her that maybe she would use 50 a year. (That was figuring high even with mailing out annual Christmas cards.) <u>Making this about Mom and not about what I wanted</u>, I asked her if there were any labels that she didn't like the print.

She said that she didn't like those that abbreviated her name just using her initials or ones with really small print. So, I pulled all of those out of the pile and asked her if I could take them home to cut up.

I asked her if there were any address labels that she didn't like the picture on the label. She pulled ones that she didn't like. I didn't nag her that she still had hundreds of address labels.

Just getting to this point took more than one visit. Even though I was a hoarder, and could see that she would only use a fraction of the address labels that she was keeping, I had to go slow with Mom; I had to work within <u>her</u> comfort level which is what you need to do with your loved one—you need to work within <u>their</u> comfort level.

In my mind, I had to celebrate small successes. I thanked Mom for going through her labels. I praised her for what she got rid of. When it was time for me to go home, I took hundreds of address labels home to cut up and throw away. Since that time, Mom has gotten more labels every week or every few weeks. Every so often we'd go through them, again, and she'd agree to let some more go. Now, sometimes Mom will surprise me by just putting some address labels in "my bag" for me to take home and cut up. Even though Mom still has more address labels than she could use in her lifetime, what she has left she likes and her pile is manageable. She feels good that she let go of what she did. I worked within her comfort level and her time tolerance. When she reached her time tolerance, she got grumpy and could not make any more decisions—it was too much for her. So, we'd stop for the day.

If you try this with your loved one, <u>asking</u> before you go through their address labels <u>together</u>, remember to keep your mouth shut when your loved one still keeps more labels than they will ever use in their lifetime. Celebrate their successes! Tell them that you are impressed that they got rid of what they did. Reinforce their positive behavior. Remember, downsizing their address labels may cause them anxiety; especially at first. By starting small, your loved one can build in their success and should be more receptive to downsizing other clutter later.

<u>Batteries</u>: Most likely your loved one has lots of batteries lying around that they don't know if they are still good or not.

Before you talk to your loved one about working on their batteries, find out where they can be dropped off. Batteries are toxic and should never be just tossed in the trash.

Your loved one is agreeable to work on batteries, today, and you have already gathered them up and sorted them into what type of battery they are; AAA, AA, C, D, etc. Your loved one has already agreed that it's frustrating to try to use a flashlight and it doesn't work and that you can recycle all of the batteries that don't work. Just keep up pleasant communication with your loved one as you try out their batteries in flashlights and other items that take that particular battery. Batteries to go are put in one box and your loved one picks a location to store all of the remaining good batteries.

When you are done with the project, thank them for all <u>they</u> accomplished today. When you leave, take the batteries to donate from their home.

<u>Book Hoarding</u>: This is my hoarding item of choice. Probably surprising to you, even though I hoard several categories of items, just thinking about downsizing my thousands of books is causing my stress level to increase

and my neck muscles are so tight it's almost painful. This is probably true for your loved one too. Even though what you see is a household of cluttered junk, to them every type of hoarded item has a value of importance even though they may have never consciously thought about it.

How this is important to you. To make the quickest progress, which in your mind isn't quick enough, it's better to work on the items which have less emotional value to them. Realize that the emotional value the hoarder has to an item has nothing to do with its monetary value. It might be easier for me to get rid of a piece of furniture than a garage sale book.

> We are not dealing with logic; we are dealing with emotional attachments.

How did I get to this point of over a thousand books? Garage sales. Church sales. Thrift shops. Almost never, except for maybe Sudoku books at a dollar store, do I ever purchase new books. Usually when I get to a Garage Sale or to a Church Sale, I get so excited I have to restrain myself from running.   "My juices are flowing!" Say a person has a box of books and there might be one or two of the books that really interests me. I will try to convince them that I will help them out, if the price is low enough, by taking all of their books off their hands. Part of the excitement is the thrill of making a great deal. So, now I have a box of books. When I'm home going through the books, I feel like a child on Christmas morning! I'm able to go through the books and get rid of a few types of books that I don't really care for. But, since I got books really cheap, there's a lot more of them that I keep because I might like them. So, instead of keeping two books, I might now keep two dozen books. This pattern is repeated over and over again.   After I go through the books, my thrill and excitement is gone. Your loved one might not have my exact pattern. For them they might not purchase used books at all; for them they might only buy new books. Whatever it is, books bring comfort, adventure, and escape from the stresses of life. If your loved one is like me, they like the feel of holding books in their hands and don't want E-books. So unless you ask them first, most likely if you gave them a present of a tablet with E-books on it, they probably won't use it.

How to help your book hoarder. (This section was so stressful for me that I had to work on other sections and come back to it.) Most likely your loved one has books stacked here and there or shoved into boxes all over their house and garage and perhaps even in a storage unit.

If you pressure your loved one and they feel that you are disrespecting them or are being judgmental, they will close up and your helping sessions has ended. Depending on how bad you treat them in <u>their</u> eyes, it might trigger them to go on a binge hoarding session after you leave. This is not about you; it's about them.

You really are going to have to honor their time tolerance level and quit when they have reached <u>their</u> time tolerance limit.

Ask your loved one if they want to help you gather up the books or if they just want to tell you where they are and you gather them up. You have stacks of books. You can put them in alphabetical order first or sort by category, first, and then work on one category putting them in alphabetical order. A category could be: pets, crafts, nonfiction mysteries or romances, religious, gardening; whatever categories they collect.

Most likely you will need many, many marked boxes. As our sort gets more specific, you can cross off what's in one box and relabel it with a new name. If your boxes are all of the same size with flaps that close, you'll be able to stack the boxes.

Some grocery stores set out milk and egg boxes which are excellent for sorting projects. If they don't set out boxes, ask the manager if they can start saving boxes for you.

Honor your loved one's time tolerance and thank them for what _they_ have done today. Stack the boxes in the garage or out of the way.

As I told you, I have thousands of books. I have two short bookcases with nicer cookbooks on the shelves. In the book room two entire sides of the room are floor to ceiling homemade shelving with books either sorted by category or favorite authors are just sorted by the author's name. Then in my bedroom I have five nice bookcases and another small bookcase that are mostly stacked two books deep. There's still a few boxes of books that I need to empty onto the shelves so I know what I have. I have already removed the duplicates and donated them.

What I'm doing and what you need to ask your loved one is which books they don't really care about anymore. Ask them if you can pull them to donate so others can enjoy them. When you are done for the day, thank them for all that they accomplished today. When you leave, take the boxes to donate from their home.

Repeat the process on your next visit(s). Since they probably will want to look at or read most of the books, accept that. Books are meant to be read.

Empower your loved one by asking them how they would like to organize their books. It could be they need bookcases or taller bookcases for their remaining books which still may be in the hundreds. Just getting their books organized into something that makes sense to your loved one will increase the chances that they will keep books off of the counters, floors, and other surfaces.

CDs and Cassette Hoarding: I know that you are in shock that anybody would keep any cassettes. There still are cassette collectors and they are not necessarily hoarders. If your loved one collects both CDs and cassettes, ask them if they would rather look at their CDs or cassettes today. Empower them to make the decision. The basic way you deal with CDs and cassettes is the same. After you complete going through CDs, go through their cassettes on a future visit.

How to help your CD (or cassette) hoarder. Your loved one has already agreed to look through either their CDs or cassettes. They make the decision on which one to work on today. Gather them together and sort according to singer's or group's name. If you have duplicates, show them both to your hoarder and then ask them to pick which one they want to keep. Put one in the marked keep box and ask them if you can put the duplicate one in the marked donate box. Then ask your loved one which of the artists or groups they don't really like anymore. Ask them if it would be okay to put them in the other box. If they have reached their time tolerance, mark and date another box that you will go through later. Put the remaining CDs (or cassettes) in there and go through the box next time. Set that box in the garage or in another area. The next visit, when your loved one is fresh, they might be more receptive to get rid of more CDs and cassettes. When you are through with one group; i.e. CDs, then you can repeat the process with cassettes. When you leave for the day, take all of the recycle, donate, and remove (throw out) items. Thank your loved one for all that <u>they</u> got done today. When both CDs and cassettes have been downsized, and you are ready to leave, thank your loved one for all <u>they</u> got done today. Praise them on completing one project.

<u>Cloth Bag Hoarding</u>: A lot of events and/or businesses give away or sell cloth bags. Ask your cloth bag hoarder if it's okay to work on their cloth bags, today.

Some bags are more useful than others. Some are thin at the bottom and are only good to carry a notebook or a few papers in them. Others expand at the bottom and are frequently used by non-hoarders, too, to put their groceries in at the grocery or other store so that they don't have to use plastic bags which do not decompose. At least this item, in your mind, has some use.

Gather up all of the cloth bags. Keep up a relaxed conversation on other subjects while you try to sort the bags into sizes with the writing facing up.

Ask your loved one if they feel good when they are able to help others. Ask them if they want to help others by donating just the bags that they don't want any more.

Ask your loved one which ones that they really don't like and pull them and place in your box to go. Ask them which ones they actually use and pull them and place them in a pile to keep. (They might not actually use any—yet.)

Remaining expandable bags. This might be a little harder for you, but keep the frustration out of your voice. If they still have quite a few expandable bags, ask them if they would like to pick three or four out to use at the grocery store. Put all of those bags into one of the bags and before you leave, today, put them in their trunk. If you live in a part of the country where you wear winter gloves, mittens, and scarves, ask them if they would like to pick out one of the expandable bags to use for their gloves, mittens, and scarves (which will be discussed below).   Other uses for the bags could be to hold store bags or other collections.

If you don't think that anybody would be interested in the bags, if you donate them, there are many bag-your-own grocery stores.   Ask the manager if they allow you to leave bags for others to use.   Cram all of the bags, to be donated, into one or more of the expandable bags.

When you have completed this project, thank them for all that <u>they</u> accomplished today. Praise them for completing this project.   When you leave, take the box to donate from their home.

<u>Coupon Hoarding</u>:   If your loved one is a coupon hoarder, they will either have stacks of cut-out coupons and/or still keep the coupon flyers with coupons that they didn't cut out. Ask your coupon hoarder if it's okay to work on their coupons, today.   Then gather up all of the coupons and coupon flyers. Keep up a relaxed conversation on other subjects while you sort the cut out coupons manufacture and store coupons into expired and non-expired coupons.

Whenever you ask your loved one a question, <u>always</u> phrase the question so that the desired answer is yes. That way, when you ask if you can donate or recycle an item, hopefully, they will be more receptive to automatically say yes.

Show the expired coupons to your loved one. Nicely explain that these coupons can never be used again and since they cannot, is it okay for you to recycle the coupons. If they agree, then put the coupons into a bag to take with you to recycle. If they balk, ask them nicely, if there is a reason for keeping their expired coupons. (Using the word "if" instead of "why" sounds less judgmental to your loved one.) Listen to their answer.   Mom will allow me to recycle her expired coupons except for one particular brand of expired store coupon. I just keep that coupon and take the rest of the expired coupons home to recycle them.

Usually in the Sunday newspaper there is one or two packets of coupons which have coupons such as $1 off of a particular brand of ice cream. Some coupon hoarders, which include me, will save coupon packets in case they need to go back to cut out a particular coupon—which I have done several times.

Ask your loved one if you can recycle the packets of coupons that they have already gone through. If they say yes, consider that one of your blessings for the day. Most likely, they will balk. At that point you have a choice of whether to just find a zone or area to store the packets of coupons until they totally expire or you take the time to go through the expired packets now. Whether decision you make, pull out the packets of coupons which have a month at the top. Generally, these coupons are only good that month. Share with your loved one that the packets of coupons that have months on them, and show them a packet several months old that has expired. Ask them if it's okay if you recycle all of these expired packets.

When your loved one goes to the grocery store with their coupons, ask them how they organize their coupons. Do not be surprised if your female hoarder just shoves the coupons loosely into their purse. If this is your hoarder, then it's probably happened at the store that they grab their stacks of coupons, to pull out a coupon, and they all drop onto the floor.

Great coupon holders are checkbook covers. You can probably get one or two free checkbook covers at your or your loved one's bank.

Ask your loved one if you picked up free checkbook covers, would they be willing to put their coupons inside of them. If they say yes, that's great!

Now we all have ideas on how things should be organized. What's logical for you might not be logical for your hoarder. If you devise a system that they don't understand soon your female coupon hoarder will have their loose coupons stuffed back in their purse again.

Ask your hoarder how they would like their coupons organized—and respect their wishes. If they say they don't know or don't care (which they really do, but don't know what they want), you could make a couple of suggestions.

If you have two checkbooks, you could ask them if they would rather have one of them for food that they eat and the other checkbook cover for non-food items OR have one for coupons that you are going to use today and the other coupons separated, on each side, by food items and non-food items. (Food items also includes beverages and candy. Non-food items also include pet food.)

Now ask your loved one if they would rather have the coupons in expiration date order or separated in some way. Whatever they say, honor _their_ system. Praise them for all that _they_ accomplished today.

The system I use, is that I use one checkbook cover. I have several sections separated by slips of paper because they make it visually easier for me to find what I'm looking for. When I first open the cover are the coupons I want to use that day or to alert me that I want to use other coupons before they expire. (The date on this group doesn't matter.) Behind this are coupons that expire this month separated by food coupons and non-food coupons. In the next section are food and beverage coupons that expire next month or later in date order with the coupons in the front the coupons that expire first. The last section are the non-food coupons which also expire next month or later in date order with the coupons in the front the coupons that expire first. Near the end of each month I try to go through the expiring coupons to see if there are some that I want to use before they expire. After a new month starts, I can easily pull out the expired coupons, recycle them, and move the new month expiring coupons to the section for coupons expiring this month.   It sounds like a lot of work, but really it's quite efficient and actually saves time in the long run; especially when I can do this when watching tv.

Then ask your loved one for their opinion. Ask them if they were to save packets of coupons until they expire, how they could be organized so that they use them. If they don't know you could share with them what a fellow hoarder does and see if they are willing to try that. What works for me is I keep a file folder loose in a certain area of my bedroom. Every week, after I cut out the coupons I might use, I take the remaining packets and put them in a file folder which is lying on its side with the most current packet on top. Periodically I pull out the file folder, turn it upside down and while watching tv. I go through the packets pulling sheets of coupons that are expired on both sides.   It works for me and keeps the coupon packets organized and it's easier for me to go through them to pull and recycle the outdated sheets of coupons.

<u>Envelope Hoarding</u>: In my case I bought too many envelopes on sale because they all weren't in one place. Now they are kept in a zone, which means in one area. I can visually see that I don't need any more envelopes so I don't buy more new envelopes. That pretty much solved my envelope hoarding. Mom hoards other envelopes. Mom is on all sorts of junk mail and non-profit mailing lists. She lived through the Great Depression. So when she receives junk mail or solicitations for donations, they generally also include an envelope. When that envelope is white, with no writing on it, Mom will keep it. Not so much anymore, but she used to also keep the return envelopes with writing on them too. In those envelopes she puts coupons or small scraps of paper.

How to help your loved one who hoards envelopes. Ask your loved one if you can look at all of their envelopes to see what they have. This includes any type of envelope to include new and used mailing envelopes and even bubble-wrap envelopes. Have your loved one help you sort the envelopes into categories such as: new small envelopes, new #10 business envelopes, new colored envelopes, new mailing envelopes, and new bubble-wrap envelopes.   Have another pile for used envelopes. Include in this pile the free white advertisement envelopes that businesses and non-profit organizations include in their mailings.

While you are sorting the envelopes, keep up a positive conversation on any topic besides their hoarding or their envelopes.

At some point you tell your loved one that you need their opinion. You are respecting their thoughts so they will be more receptive to them. Ask them what would work for them to hold their envelopes and where would they like all of their envelopes to be stored. (For me, my envelopes are kept in one zone or area. At a sale, I bought quite a few see-through plastic containers with lids; some were shoe box sized and others were larger with lids. Regular envelopes fit in the shoe box container and the #10 business envelopes fit in another container with a lid.)

Remember, although the containers work for me—which means that it was logical to me, it might not be logical for your loved one. If it is not logical to them, they won't do it—or do it for very long.

Say your loved one says that they want all of their envelopes to go into a drawer, which is full with other stuff. Be agreeable and empty the drawer into a box or bag, for now, and mark the box or bag either where it came from or what's in it. Set it aside to deal with later; most likely on the next visit. Actually since the drawer can only hold so many envelopes that might actually help you, but more on that later.

Most likely your loved one has really old never-used envelopes. Pull out all of the ones that are stuck closed and put them all in one pile. Pull out all of the really yellowed envelopes and put them all in one pile near the stuck-envelope pile. The usable new envelopes are stacked in piles according to their size.

Show them first the stuck envelopes and explain that because they are stuck together, they are unusable. Ask them if it's okay for you to recycle them. Pull out one of the really yellowed envelopes and ask them if they would rather receive a yellowed envelope or a white envelope. They should say white envelopes. Ask them if it's okay to recycle them. For whatever envelopes that they are willing to recycle, put them immediately in a bag and put by your pile to take with you to recycle when you leave for the day.

If your loved one thinks they will use containers, which they probably don't have, box the envelopes and mark the box so you don't forget and have to resort it later.

If your loved one's time tolerance has expired, tell them that you are just going to box up the remaining envelopes so you both can look at them during your next visit. (Be sure to mark the box or bag and date it, which will save you time later.)

Before leaving, praise them for all that <u>they</u> got accomplished today (even though its way less than you had wanted).

During your next visit, nicely with a good tone of voice, go over any envelopes—and other will-decide-on-later items from previous sorts. If they agree to donate (or recycle or otherwise get rid of) some more of their items, immediately put them in your box or bag to take with you when you leave today.

Now it's their used envelopes which also includes blank or printed on envelopes from advertisers and non-profit organizations. Sort the envelopes according to their kind: new and used large envelopes and new and used bubble-wrap envelopes, (any envelope larger than #10 business envelope), preprinted and blank envelopes from advertisers and non-profit organizations. It doesn't matter which sorted pile you start from.

Let's say you start with the advertisers and non-profit organization envelopes. Show them the two stacks. Ask them if it would be okay, since they have a lot of non-printed envelopes, if the printed envelopes can be recycled. (To most hoarders, recycling or donating the item is better than throwing the item away.) If they are agreeable, then put them in a box or bag to go with you when you leave for the day. If they have reached their time tolerance, and balk, then ask them if it's okay to, instead, put them in a marked box or bag, and put it in the garage for now. Then next visit, ask again, nicely, until they are agreeable.

Most, if not all of the advertisement white envelopes, have windows cut out of them. Nicely, ask them what they plan to use the envelopes with the windows cut out of them for. Ask them if it would be okay to keep three of them and donate (or recycle) the rest of them. If they say yes to donate, then you will put them in a clear baggie to donate. If they say they need more envelopes saved, don't question them; just ask how many and, for now, keep out those extra envelopes. Either way, you are still able to reduce their hoard of white envelopes with windows in them.

If your loved one has both new and used larger envelopes and bubble-wrap envelopes, point to the new envelopes and ask them, nicely, that since they have so many nice envelopes, people would much rather receive a clean envelope than one that has been scratched out, don't they agree? If they agree, then ask them if it would be okay to recycle the used paper envelopes (after ripping out the metal closer). If they agree, then immediately put them in your box or bag that goes with you when you leave. If they disagree, then put them in a box or bag and put in the garage to deal with during a later visit.

Surprisingly, getting rid of used bubble wrap might be more difficult, so don't get defensive if their anxiety level goes up; it's not about you.

Ask them, nicely and with a good tone of voice, if they are keeping the used bubble wrap for a particular reason. (If you say "why" instead of "if", it might come across as more judgmental and their anxiety level may start to rise and you are, now, basically done sorting for the day.)

If they say that they haven't had time to cut off their address and cut it up, don't laugh or judge them. This is actually the best scenario for you. Ask them if it would be okay for you to take the envelopes and cut out and cut up their address labels. They should say yes. Put the envelopes in your bag or box to go and later cut up their address and throw the envelopes away since they cannot be recycled.

If they say that they might need the bubble wrap later, don't pull your hair out when you know that they will probably never need the bubble wrap. Keep the frustration out of your voice. Instead ask them that <u>to make it easier for you</u>, would it be okay if you cut off the front of the envelope to take home and cut up their address which will leave <u>them</u> with clean stacks of bubble wrap ready to use. The emphasis is on them and that you are helping them. If they are agreeable then either together or by yourself, their choice, the envelopes can be cut up.

Ask them where they would like to stack their clean bubble wrap. If they decide on the zone or area to keep their bubble wrap and other envelopes, they are more likely to keep the items in their zone.

<u>Food Hoarding</u>: In this section I'm talking about non-perishable food that comes in cans, bottles, and packages. (Perishable foods are talked about below.) The food hoarder has food all over their home. There usually doesn't seem to be any organization to all of the boxes, bottles, and packages of food that they have. Often they have expired food. When there is a sale, they might stockpile food; often purchasing more of the item than they can use before it expires.

If your loved one ever went hungry at some point in their life, they might have this fear of not having enough food; especially if they lived through the Great Depression. They might have vowed that they'd never go hungry again. The wrong thing to tell your loved one is that they don't have to hoard food because they have enough food to last them five years. You are disrespecting the trauma that they endured. If you've never gone to bed hungry, then you don't get it. Never tell them that you are coming over to help them organize and get rid of excess food. This will increase their anxiety. You are disrespecting them. If you take their food, even if it has expired, without their permission, you are stealing their food from them.

It will not stop their food hoarding. In fact, because you disrespected them, it might cause them to go purchase more food with money that they might not really have to spare, just because your behavior stressed them out.

Instead of telling them what you are going to do, instead ask them, nicely, if you can just help them organize their food. Reassure them, and then keep your word, that you will not take any food out of their house without their permission. When you are helping them, don't mumble, under your breath, about their mess. You may have boxes and containers in your vehicle; however, do not take them immediately into their house or their anxiety will skyrocket and they will get defensive.

Once they say yes, and don't bully them into saying yes, then when you get to their home, you can quickly access the situation. Ask them if they would rather start with the kitchen counter or the garage or one shelf in their cupboard. Empower them to make a decision. This little thing, allowing them to make even such a minor decision, is really a biggie to them. If they suggest another place to start, be agreeable to their suggestion.

Remember, their tolerance level. If it's only 15 minutes, don't start setting things out, which will take 2 hours to sort and clean up.

If they are older, you might bring a chair to the area you will be working on; otherwise, bring the items closer to them so that they don't have to be on their feet which will tire them out even faster.

My suggestion is to have a magic marker and write the expiration date on the part of the package that will be viewed when it's organized in a cabinet or on a shelf. Ask your loved one if they would like to be the one who marks the item. Ask them if it's okay to just put the month, a slash mark, and the two-digit year that the food expires. Keep your mouth shut if you find something that has expired several years ago.

If a box mix has milk or eggs in it, it should be tossed when it has expired. But do this with caution—and don't you just throw the expired

<u>food out without their permission</u>. Remember, you need to respect your loved one.

Say I was going through Mom's pantry and found a box of cake mix that had expired two years ago. I might casually say, "Mom, would it be a good thing or a bad thing if you ate some bad food and you got sick and went to the hospital?" Of course she would agree that it would be bad to get food poisoning. I might then continue with, "Food that has expired eggs and milk in it can cause people to get very sick. You want to remain healthy and not get food poisoning, right?" She doesn't want to get sick. I might keep going by saying, "Mom, to keep you from getting sick from expired eggs and milk, do I have your permission to get rid of this cake mix that has expired eggs in it?" Since I've empowered her, she should be agreeable and I've gotten her permission. At that time, I might get a box or a bag and recycle the cardboard box and put the expired cake mix package in the bag. When I leave, the expired cake mix goes to my house and into my trash so that she cannot take it out of the trash. The outer box is recycled.

We hoarders are sneaky. We have to be. Because you are stealing our food, by taking it without our permission, if you put it in our trash, after you leave, we might march out to the trash bin and retrieve the food you have taken from us. Then we will hide the food so you don't find it. <u>You have to get this—we aren't doing this to defy you. We are doing this because you took our food, without our permission.</u> This is stealing and extremely disrespectful to us. When we take the expired food, or other item, that you put in our trash can, out of the trash can, we are only retrieving what you stole from us. Even though your intent may be good, because you love us, show us your love by helping us in a way that respects and empowers us.

Let's say that today you asked your loved one and they agreed that together you could do one shelf of food. Keep your word to them; just pull one shelf's worth of items off of the shelf. While you or your loved one are marking the expiration date on the front of the package, you are also sorting the packages into expired and not expired piles. At that time, do <u>not</u> put any expired food in any trash bags or boxes; just set them aside in one pile.

You've finished marking the one shelf's worth of packages. Before putting the non-expired items back on the shelf, ask your loved one if there's any of the food items that they don't like. If they say yes, ask permission if you can donate them to a food pantry (if they aren't expired.) If they are agreeable, pull those packages and put them in a box or bag to go. Make sure that if you say they are going to a food pantry that the food ends up at the food pantry.

Realize that, today, you might only get some cans and packages marked with the expiration date before your loved one's time tolerance has been exhausted. That's okay. It took your loved one more than a few days to get the collection of food that they have. You need to be content with the baby steps of progress that your loved has just done. Remember, this is stressful to them. If you have an attitude, their stress level skyrockets and their tolerance time will be significantly reduced.

Before putting the dated food back on the shelves, ask your loved one where they want them placed on the shelf. Put the packages that haven't expired back on the shelf, sorted by type of item; i.e. all green bean cans are together. Have the cans that expire the soonest closest to the front of the shelf so that they are eaten first. I've read that most foods that don't have milk or eggs in them can be safely eaten for at least one year past the Best By date. If you have packages that are clearly outdated, you tell your loved one that these items are past their safe date to eat and will they give you permission to remove them so that they don't get sick. If yes, then put them in your box or bag and remove them from their house when you leave. Since they are probably at or past their tolerance level already, their anxiety level is rising. Realize and respect that. If they balk, then nicely ask them if you can put the expired packages in the box and put the box in the garage. Thank them for all that <u>they</u> did today. For them it was a biggie.

> How you word sentences may be the difference between success and frustration. For items that will be thrown away, <u>don't</u> say: throw away or get rid of. Instead say remove, which sounds less final.

On your next visit, when they are fresh, you can ask them again if you have their permission to remove the cans in the garage that have expired and are unsafe to eat. If they agree, then immediately take the box to your vehicle.

If they, again, balk, say nothing, and let the topic drop. Next visit, ask again—nicely.

The cycle starts all over again. You ask and don't tell. You respect their wishes even though you don't agree with their decision about hanging on to expired food. Only try to do enough sorting that you think you can finish before their time tolerance level is reached. Celebrate and don't be frustrated by their baby steps.

By now, some time has passed. With your loved one's permission, you've gone through their cupboards and their packages are marked with the expiration date. If you get the grocery ads you know what's on sale. If your loved one purchases canned corn when it's on sale, you might ask them if they've seen this week's grocery ad. You might casually, and nonjudgmentally, remind them that they don't need any more corn, but they might pick up one or two cans of peas (if their stash of peas is dwindling enough that they could get a couple of cans of peas that they should be able to eat before they expire.) That way, they still feel good about getting a bargain—peas on sale and, hopefully, remember that they have enough corn.

Then periodically you both can go through their pantry and do any maintenance—sorting and marking that's necessary—with your loved one's permission, of course.

Thank them for what <u>they</u> got accomplished today. When they have finished this project praise them.

<u>Hotel Soaps and Shampoos and Other Hotel Freebie Hoarding</u>: We cannot help it; if it's free, we take it home with us. Ask your loved one if, today, we can look at their hotel freebies. Empower them by asking if they would rather help you collect the freebies or if they just want to tell you where they are and you get them. Sort into used and unused soaps, shampoos, conditioners, hand lotion, shower caps, and other freebies that they have collected over the years.

Ask them if there are any of the freebies that they won't use. If they were to say shower caps, ask them if they would rather donate them to a homeless shelter, a women's shelter, or to a charity. If they are receptive, bag or box up what they are willing to donate.

Ask them that since they are on a roll, are there other items that they would be willing to help others with by donating. If they are receptive, put those items in the donate bag or box.

Ask them nicely, that since they have so many soaps (or list the freebie item) left, would they be willing to help others out by donating at least some of them. If yes, put them in your donate box. Repeat with every freebie item. Hopefully, but not necessarily, they have whittled down their freebies down to a more manageable size. If their hoard is still high in one or more of the items, you could nicely ask them if they could reduce the item down to ____, (where you pick a number that should at least be three). If they agree, put more freebies in the donate box.

Now to the partially used freebie items. Most hoarders do not like to waste items; no matter what it is. This is our reality, so you need to work with us here. Remember, if you start nagging or complaining, we are done downsizing for at least today and your attitude may send us into a hoarding buying frenzy. You don't want the downsizing to stop—or their clutter to increase.

You should ask your hoarder what they want to do with the used freebies. They might say to throw them out, although it's doubtful. Look on the bottom to see if the containers are recyclable. If they are, you could remind them that the containers can be recycled. This might make them more receptive to removing (getting rid of) them.

Make this a benefit for them. Ask them if they would like you to combine the partial bottles so that they would be easier to use. This might help. You could ask if it was okay if you took care of the empty bottles to get them out of their way. (It's better to not say throw out. That's not a good word for hoarders.) Respect their answer—either way.

Now, together, you have downsized what your loved one was willing to do. Always thank them for what <u>they</u> accomplished, today, and take the donate items and the recycle items when you leave.

Ask them how they would like to store the freebies that they want to keep. Accept or suggest alternatives, but keep your voice calm and nonjudgmental. They might see that they have too many and may be willing to donate more of the freebies. If not, then assist them in their suggestion on how to store the freebies.

Thank them for what <u>they</u> got accomplished today. When they have finished this project praise them.

<u>Magazine Hoarding</u>: I am a magazine hoarder. This year I donated magazines that dated back to the 1970s. What helps me is that our library has a table where people donate their magazines and where others eagerly snatch them up. Otherwise, I would have recycled the magazines; but I feel better that others can enjoy them too. As a researcher magazine hoarder, I was able to go through hundreds of magazines, ripping out pages that interested me. Even though I may never look at what I ripped out, it was the only way for me to thin the stacks down. I have probably gone through 60 - 70% of the boxes that contain magazines even though I probably have over 100 magazines left to go through.

How to help your loved one who hoards magazines. This one might be more frustrating for you. In your mind, the information is outdated and there's no reason to save the magazines. If you really want to help your hoarder, you need to not nag or complain or threaten your hoarder or the extra anxiety you are causing them will probably send them into an additional hoarding frenzy. Still respecting them and their tolerance time, ask them if you can just gather their magazines.

> Reassure them that you won't get rid of any magazines against their will.

Keep a steady conversation going, talking about positive subjects and not their clutter or their magazines.

Sort all of the magazines into piles by the name of the magazine. Then put all of the magazines in date order. Since your loved one probably picks up magazines where they find them, most likely there are duplicates. If you find duplicates, show both of them to your loved one. Tell them that these are exactly the same magazine and ask them which one they want to keep. They will pick one and put that in the stack and place the other one in a pile. After you have gone through the magazines, remind your loved one that the one pile is duplicates; they are exactly the same magazine that they saved in a separate pile. Ask them if it's okay for you to recycle (or donate) the duplicates. If they say yes, then put them in your pile to go when you leave. If they balk, then don't argue with them. Ask them, instead, if you can move the duplicates to the garage. Be sure to mark the box or bag with the word duplicates. Then the next time you visit, ask the same questions about the duplicates. If their time tolerance has expired, then you can box the magazines and stack the boxes.

Before you leave, write down the name of each magazine name. Most likely they will have a variety of magazines. On your next visit, in a calm voice, tell them that last visit you both sorted their magazines according to the name of the magazine and then you both put them in date order. Take out the piece of paper and ask them if there's any of the magazines that they really don't even like anymore. If they are able to name one or more magazines that they really don't care about, ask them if it would be okay if you recycle or donate those magazines so others can enjoy them. If yes, box or bag them up and follow through to recycle (or donate) them like you promised them. Realize that for magazine hoarders, getting rid of any magazines is a big deal. Praise them for recycling or donating their magazines.

Then, with the list in your hands, ask them if any of the magazines are ones that they just look at the pictures. If they say yes, ask them if it would be okay if you get those magazines out of the boxes. Ask them if they would be willing to look through a few of them, at their leisure, before you visit again. They should be agreeable to at least humoring you by saying yes. If they go through at least one magazine, praise them. Now the moment of truth. Ask them some unrelated questions where the answer should be yes. Then ask them if it's okay to recycle (or donate) the look-and-get-rid of magazines that they've gone through. If yes, put them in your pile to go. If no, and it might be, take a pen and put their initials on the top right corner to signify that they have already gone through that magazine. Keep talking about unrelated events where the answers to the questions are yes. Ask them if it's okay if you put the magazines that they read in the garage.

During your next visit, while they are still fresh and not at their time tolerance, yet, you remind them that last visit they had already read these magazines. Show them the marking on the top right corner of the magazine. Remind them that last time <u>we</u> marked these to show that you had gone through them. Ask again, if it would be okay to recycle (or donate) these magazines that they've already gone through.

Once they are through with one type of magazine, line through that title of that magazine on their list. Praise them for their accomplishment. While they are happy with your praise, ask them which magazine on the list would be the next easy for them to read.

At some point, there will be information that your loved one will want to keep and that's one reason that they have kept that magazine. Ask them if they would be willing to rip out the article they want from the magazine, save it, and recycle (or donate) the rest of the magazine. If they are receptive, keep repeating the process.

If there are one or more magazines that they really love, and don't want to depart with, accept that, and be thrilled that they have reduced their magazine hoarding by a huge percentage.

<u>Makeup Hoarding</u>: Your loved one may have collected makeup and perfume since they were a teenager. Ask, today, if your loved one is willing to look at their makeup. Gather all of their makeup into one area separating it into categories such as lipstick, tweezers, clippers,

emery files, powder, eyeliner, perfume, and whatever other categories your loved one may have.

Ask them if they see anything that they just don't like or use anymore. Ask them if you can put it in the bag.   Unless the item is new or clippers or tweezers, it will need to be thrown out and cannot be donated. Pick a category and go through each item to see how much more of that item they are willing to put in the bag. If makeup or lipstick looks all dried up, show them that it is unusable and ask if you can put it in the bag.

For tweezers and clippers, ask them which one's they like the best and put that in the keep pile. For multiple items of the same thing, ask them if they could only pick two tweezers or two clippers, which ones would they pick. Ask if it's okay to keep the ones that they really like and to donate the others. Ask your loved one which tweezers and clippers don't work as well as you want them too. Ask them that since they don't like these tweezers and clippers if it's okay to donate them.

Most likely your loved one will have opened and unopened items still in their packages. If they want to keep both the opened and unopened item of the same thing, nicely ask them where you could store all of the unopened items so they are kept all together. You might ask them if they would use a plastic shoe box with a top to keep them conveniently in one place.

Thank them for all that <u>they</u> got accomplished today. Once they finish the project, praise them.

<u>Medical Supply Hoarding</u>: A medical supply hoarder has lots of medical supplies to include cough syrups, over-the-counter medications, ointments, vitamins and supplements, Band-Aids, wraps, as well as other medical-related items. Ask your loved one if, today, you could look at their medical supplies. Bring all of their medical supplies to one area and sort according to category; all of the ointments together, all of the Band-Aids together, etc.

Most likely some of the ointments, over-the counter medications, and cough syrups are years past their expiration date.

Ask your loved one that if they were sick and they took medicine or used ointment on it, would they be upset if it didn't work. They should answer yes. Show them all of the medical supplies that have passed their expiration date. Ask them that if you recycle the outer cardboard wrappers, is it okay, for their health and safety, to remove just the outdated items. Put them in the bag to take with you. If they balk, ask them if we purchase usable replacement items, would they be willing to put the outdated items in the bag. If they are receptive, make a list of items to purchase and next visit remind them of what they said and replace the outdated items with current replacement items.

Do the same thing with all of their vitamins, supplements, and other dated items that you hadn't discussed before.

Now you should just have non-dated items left. Say they have several wraps and braces. At the most they should only need two of each. (I asked a non-hoarder if two was a reasonable amount to work towards and she agreed and she has bad knees and ankles.) You might ask your loved one which are the best two wraps in the pile. Pull them out. Remind them that since these two are the best, they could help others if they would donate the rest. Do the same with the braces. Be receptive to their wishes because they have probably reached their time tolerance.

Band-Aids. Most likely your hoarder has opened and unopened boxes of Band-Aids. Ask your loved one if there are any of the Band-Aids that they don't like. Ask your loved one if you can put the Band-Aids in the bag to donate. Ask your loved one if you can put the unopened Band-Aids in the plastic container with the other unopened Band-Aids. Thank your loved one for all that <u>they</u> accomplished today and take the bags to donate and throw away with you when you leave.

<u>Newspaper Hoarding</u>: I am a researcher and a newspaper hoarder. Yes, I know that the information is old news. In our minds, that's okay. In our minds something might interest us later, so we keep the newspapers. It doesn't matter that we could get the information faster on the internet.

How to help your loved one who hoards newspapers. This hoarding is going to test your patience. You have to remember that if you nag or threaten your loved one, their anxiety level will skyrocket and this will be the end of their downsizing today and will most likely send them on a hoarding binge to calm them down.

Remember, it's about them and not you. Suggestion, some grocery stores set out egg and milk boxes for the public to take. If they don't, ask if they could save you some. Newspapers fit into them nicely and keeps them from falling all over the place.

Most likely, if your loved one hoards newspapers, they will be all over the house and most likely intermixed with other papers, such as bills.

Before you bring any boxes in, ask your loved one if it's okay if, together, that we collect the newspapers just to put them in one place. Reassure your loved one that you aren't going to do anything with the newspapers without their consent. This should keep their anxiety level fairly calm.

Ask your loved one, in a calm, nonjudgmental voice, <u>to make it easier for them</u>, if you have their permission to recycle all of the outdated ads. If they say yes, you can pull all of the outdated ads and place them in a pile.

As you are collecting all of the newspapers, ask your loved one if there's any section of the newspaper that they don't read. If they were to tell you, for example, that they don't read the sports section, ask them if it's okay if you pulled out all of the sports sections to recycle since they don't read that section anyways. If they are receptive, then all of the sports sections can be pulled and put in a pile and later a box or bag to recycle. If they say that there is one page that's in the sports section that they read, ask them if you can pull that page out for them to look at later, and recycle the rest of that section. It should be okay for them. (In the sports section, they may have one or more pages that are not sports related.)

Ask your loved one if it's okay for you to go get boxes to neatly stack the newspapers in. They should say yes. If they do, gather up the newspaper sections that they agreed that you could recycle and take them to your vehicle at the same time you are getting the boxes.

Most likely their time tolerance has expired and they are getting more tense and anxious. Before filling the boxes neatly with all of the piles of newspapers, ask them in there are any sections that they are able to quickly go through. If they name one or more sections, ask them if it would be okay if you keep some of those sections out so that they can look at them before your next visit.

At this point, just neatly put all of the piles of newspapers into the boxes, without mumbling under your breath or complaining. Ask your loved one where they would like you to stack the boxes until your next visit.

To you it might not feel like you've accomplished anything, but to your loved one, today has been a huge accomplishment.

Before leaving, praise your love one for what <u>they</u> did today. Always leave a hoarder's house on a happy note!

> When hoarders are feeling less stressed, they are more likely to work on downsizing.

<u>Outdated Medication Hoarding</u>: Outdated medication either might not work in the way it's supposed to, work in an unsafe manner, or become more potent. You might ask your loved one if it's okay if, today, together we go

through their meds. If they are agreeable, then pull all of their prescription and non-prescription medications. Also, if there's time, pull creams and sunscreen. Ask your loved one if there are any medications that they don't take anymore. Set them aside. Any medications that are expired put in the same pile. Do the same for outdated creams and sunscreen. Once you are done, ask your loved one that if they were sick and they took their meds and they didn't work, would that be a bad thing. They would say yes. Then tell them that the one pile has expired meds and they might not work when they needed them to do. Ask them if you can remove them so that their health isn't in jeopardy. If they say yes, immediately bag them up to take them with you when you leave. If they balk, then accept their wishes, but ask if you can put the expired meds in a bag and put in the garage. Then the next visit, when they are fresh, ask the same questions. Once they say yes, remove the bag from the house. Many pharmacies have drug drop-off sites where <u>you</u> can drop off the outdated drugs.

Thank them for all that <u>they</u> got accomplished today. Once they finish the project, praise them.

<u>Paper Hoarding</u>: Situation: Mail comes in. Lot of it is unsolicited advertisements or what everybody calls junk mail. Often the paper hoarder is afraid of throwing away something that is or might someday be important. So it gets stacked up on the table or counter or other surface area where the paper hoarder puts their mail. Unfortunately, important paperwork, such as bills get mixed up with the junk mail and may be forgotten and the bill becomes overdue and late fees accumulate.

As we have discussed, clutter often worsens with age. My mother is 92 years old—and a hoarder. Junk mail has evolved so that a lot of it looks like important paperwork. So, Mom saves this mail. She's also on a lot of junk-mail mailing lists. Often these advertisements might put a teaser trinket in them such as mailing labels or a pad of paper. So she saves the entire advertisement. Tuesdays are Mom's Day when I usually go to her apartment and we run errands, go to doctor's appointments, and I get her groceries for her. If I see a stack of mail on her table, I <u>ask her</u> if we can go through the mail. I <u>ask her permission</u> if I can open all of the letters for her. I <u>ask her</u> if I can recycle advertisements. If she says yes, then I put those papers in one pile. If she says no, I put them in another pile. I don't judge her; I accept her decision. Then, so she cannot change her mind, I take all of the junk mail home to shred.

Remember, what seems logical for you, might not be logical for your loved one. Ask your loved one their opinion on how they think they can tackle their stack of mail. You are showing them respect by asking their opinion and not telling them what they must do. Ask them if they had two baskets, if they could throw bills in one basket and everything else in the other basket. Ask them if they wanted to go out and buy the baskets or not. You are empowering them and they are more likely to do it if it makes sense to them. For some paper hoarders, baskets might work for them. For others, they might suggest that they would rather use those paper sorters that they have at office supply stores. Great! Whatever system they will use to tame their clutter is the objective here. If you try to force them to use a clutter-reducing idea, and it doesn't make sense to them, it won't work and they won't use it at all or for very long.

When you visit with them, you can see if they are using the baskets. If they aren't, gently talk to them about it. If they are using the baskets, you can ask them if it would be okay if we sit down at the table and write out the bills. With Mom I write out the check. Mom signs it and puts the stamp and address label on the envelope.   Then sometimes I take the envelopes and personally mail her bills.

If your loved one is using the baskets, when you visit you can ask your loved one if it is okay if you look at what's in the other basket, which is the junk-mail basket. Expect some of the letters won't even be opened. Always ask permission to open the envelopes. Then ask permission if you can take certain envelopes home to shred. If they say balk, don't argue with them. Say nothing; just put that envelope back in the junk-mail basket. By respecting their wishes, even though you don't agree with their decision, may make it easier, next time, for them to part with more junk mail. Remember, celebrate their baby steps. For hoarders, getting rid of something that they hoard, is stressful.   It doesn't matter if you don't think that it has any value; it has emotional value to your loved one.

Thank them for all that <u>they</u> got accomplished today.   Once they finish the project, praise them.

<u>Pen and Pencil Hoarding</u>: This category would also include markers, crayons, and craft paints. Say your loved one has hundreds of pens and pencils; because they have gotten them for free at banks and other places. It's not that they have collected them as part of vacation; it's because they were free. If you know where your loved one stashes their pens and pencils, ask if you can pull them all out to look at them. As you are just making conversation, make two piles; one pencils and one pens. Ask your loved one if you can test all of the pens. Using scrap paper, which I'm sure they have tons of on hand, just sit and test each pen putting the dried up ink pens in one pile and the pens that are still good in another pile. If your loved one wants to help, let them. Keep the conversation light. When you are through testing all of the pens, ask them if they've ever grabbed a pen and got frustrated when it didn't work. They should answer yes. You can point to the pens and tell them that these pens are dried up and will never work again. Ask them if you can get rid of them, which is better than saying that you want to throw them away. Throwing away sounds so final to a hoarder and might increase their anxiety. If they say yes, put them in the pile for you to take with you and throw them away. If they want to keep some of the pens

that don't work, bite your tongue and say nothing. Just say okay. If they say no, don't be offended; it's not about you. Keep your voice and especially your tone nice. Ask them if you can put them in a bag and put the ones that don't work and put in the garage. Reinsure them that you aren't throwing them away; you are just separating them from the ones that work. If they agree, put them in the bag and put them in the garage without mumbling or complaining. The next time you visit, ask again if you can get rid of just the pens that are dried up and will never work again. If they say yes, immediately remove them from their home; if no, say nothing and try again next time.

Thank them for all that <u>they</u> got accomplished today. Once they finish the project, praise them.

<u>Plastic Bag and Paper Bag Hoarding</u>: This is when your loved one saves plastic store and paper bags as well as bread bags and other plastic and paper bags.

This category is probably another category that really frustrates non hoarders. To you, the bags are trash. For some of us hoarders we reuse the bags because most of them do not break down in the landfills; especially plastic bags.

How to help your plastic bag and paper bag hoarder: Ask your loved one, nicely, if, today, we can look at their plastic and paper bags. It's going to be hard, but don't complain or mumble underneath your breath about keeping garbage or your loved one will feel disrespected and shut down and that will be the end of the downsizing session today. Depending on how much you distress your loved one, it might also send them into a hoarding-buying frenzy.

After all of the bags have been collected, sort them according to size and type of material (paper and plastic). You should have a pile of store plastic bags, store paper bags, and other bags in various sizes.

Before you tackle this project, I would contact food pantries and/or thrift shops and ask them if they need store plastic or paper bags. Some bag-your-own-grocery stores may allow you to leave bags for others to use. Also, some grocery stores have bins where you can put clean plastic bags that do not have holes in them.

Ask your loved one, nicely, if there is a reason why they are keeping so many bags. Listen to their answer. If they balk, ask them if you can put the bags in a (marked and dated) box and put the box in the garage.

Plastic bags that have had raw meat in them should NEVER be reused. Even if they are washed, they still could have bacteria on them that can make you very, very sick.

When you leave, take all of the bags with you that will be donated, recycled, or thrown in the trash. Thank them for all that <u>they</u> got accomplished today. Once they finish the project, praise them.

<u>Plastic Container Hoarding</u>: This category is different from restaurant take-out container hoarding which is discussed below. These are plastic containers with tight-fitting lids and come in an assortment of sizes and shapes. Some are square, others are rectangles, and others are circular.

How to help your plastic container hoarder: Ask your loved one if, today, we could look at their plastic containers. After you have collected up all of the containers, sort them to size. Make a pile of any extra lids or containers without lids.

Ask them if there are any plastic containers that they don't like any more or that they have trouble getting the lids off of. Ask them if you can take them with you (to donate, recycle, or throw away). Put them in a box or bag to go.

Ask them that since they have so many good containers, would it be okay to remove the containers that have either no lids or no bottoms. Ask if it would be okay to remove the stained containers. All of these containers, that they agree to remove, will go in the pile that you will take with you.

Most likely they will have old margarine and other food containers with their lids. They should also have a lot of storage containers that were purchased new at a store or used ones that were bought at garage and other sales.

Ask them if they have ever put food in a food container, such as a margarine container, and then forgot what was in it. Ask them, so that doesn't happen to them again, if you can remove all of those containers and recycle the containers. If yes, put them in your box to go.

If they balk, ask them if you can put them in a (marked and dated) box and put in the garage.

Ask them what zone they have to store their containers in. If they look at you funny, tell them that a zone is an area. (This will start their mind thinking in zones before you get to the next section. It could make the transition to zones less stressful for them.)   Look from their containers to the space. Your loved one knows that there isn't enough space for what they have. Without complaining or being sarcastic, nicely ask them if they have any suggestions on how you can help them make all of their containers fit. Listen to them.

At this point I would ask them to start pointing to the containers that they really like and ask them where on the shelf they want them. Put them on the shelf. Keep doing this, stacking like containers. If you still have containers left, ask them if it would okay for you to remove the remaining containers. If yes, put them in your box or bag. If they balk, ask them if it is okay to put them in the (marked and dated) box to be put in the garage.

When you are done, thank your loved one for what <u>they</u> got accomplished today. When you leave, take all of the containers with you that will be donated, recycled, or thrown in the trash. Once they have finished this project, praise them.

<u>Record Album Hoarding</u>: Don't groan, but are you aware that they are making record albums again?

If your loved one hoards record albums, they probably have hundreds of them. One problem is that they are so heavy. I should know; I have thousands of them. But, I announced that I'm ready to get rid of the ones I'm hoarding (and won't be listening to again.) That still leave a couple of hundred that I'm keeping that I could possibly listen to again—and that's okay.

How to help your record album hoarder. Be advised, this will most likely take many visits so if there is something else that they hoard, it may be easier to start with other items. But if today is the day that your loved one has agreed to work on record albums that translates to that today is the day that you <u>start</u> working on record albums. Since record albums tend to have memories attached to them, do not collect all of their record albums. In fact, do not collect the record albums that are near their record player;

pick record albums stashed in different parts of their home.

Ask your loved one which record albums they want to look at first. You might have to ask where they are.

You need to, in a nice voice ask your loved one if there is a reason they are collecting record albums. (Ask "if" and not "why" because why seems more judgmental.) Listen to what they say without judging them.   How they reply determines on how you respond to them.

My story. Like books, at sales if there tended to be lots of record albums I'd bid on the entire batch of them and purchase them if I could get them cheaply enough. So now I have a few hundred that I might listen to and easily have over a 1,000 record albums that need to go. If like me, your hoarder says that they might be worth something, they might. However, having said that, most of them probably aren't worth much. So I'm negotiating on what price to put on them to donate them. One non-profit thrift store sells records for really good prices. To get the most value when donating them, they have to be donated to this one store. Since the donating limit is below $500, per visit without having the records valued first, there will be many, many different trips to donate the records.

If the record album hoarding is due to the fact that your loved one thinks some records have value, then you can put different values on them when you donate them. If they refuse to donate, then you can see if they would be willing, first, to have a record dealer come to the house, while you are there, to purchase records from you. If you don't know the person, you don't know if they are giving you a fair price or not; however, you will hopefully be able to get rid of some of the records. Then, your loved one may be more receptive to donating the other stacks of record albums. (Or, if your loved one uses the internet, they can look up what albums are selling for used.

You can call or Email a record album business to see what they are looking for, first. It would probably be less anxiety producing if your loved one is not there when the buyer looks over the record albums. They might get anxious when they hear that some/most/all of the record albums aren't worth anything. They might internalize that rejection. Also, it's probably better if the record albums are boxed, with only enough records in each box, so they are easily browsed through.   Have the record album covers all going the same way so that the buyer can just quickly flip through them.

But before you even talk to a buyer or donate their record albums, your loved one needs to go through the albums. One stack at a time, you need to ask your loved one if there are any singers that they don't like. Pull them aside. The ones that they need to think about, start putting in boxes in alphabetical order. When you find duplicates, show them both of the albums. Look at the actual album to see which one looks better. Ask them which one that they would rather keep. Set the keep albums in one marked box in alphabetical order and the do something with albums in another marked box in alphabetical order. Yes, this project is going to take a long time and not many record album decisions may be made in one visit. At the end of their time tolerance, quit and thank them for <u>their</u> progress.

Resume working on records your next visit up to their time tolerance and thank <u>them</u> for their progress at the end of each sorting session. Once they finish this project praise them.

<u>Recycle Hoarding</u>: If your loved one felt the hardship of the Great Depression, they might save everything. If your loved one has bottles, cans, glass, scrap metal, and anything else that can be recycled in their house, in their garage, and/or overflowing into their yard, then they are a recycle hoarder. Their initial intent was to turn the items in for money. Now they feel overwhelmed. If their recycle hoarding has flowed out into the yard, they might get a warning or a ticket from the town they live in. If this happens to them, they will get mad and think the town is bullying them.

You have a couple of angles that you could use depending on what's important to them. Say they've been eyeing a new fishing rod. You could start a question about that fishing rod. Ask them if they had the money, would they buy the fishing rod that they had been admiring. They should say yes. (They could already have enough money to purchase the fishing rod, but may tend to not spend their money.)

You know if your loved one needs to think about things before they make a decision. If that is your loved one, then you are not going to get them to commit to anything today. Mention that you think they would love to have that fishing rod that they've been admiring. Tell them that you are willing, if they are, that you and perhaps others might be willing to help them take their recycle items (don't say junk) to turn in for money so they can purchase their fishing rod. (Call it _their_ fishing rod.) Then drop talking about it and talk about something else. The next time you see them, if they haven't mentioned it to you already, ask them if they have been thinking about _their_ fishing rod. If they say yes, then ask them if they've thought about you helping them to get their fishing rod by turning in the recycle items for cash so they can purchase _their_ fishing rod. If they agree then, together, figure out how to tackle the project. (Call it a project and not junk.)

Once you have the recycle items off of the property, tell your loved one that you need their opinion. Ask them what system would work best for them _to make it easier for them_ to organize their recycle items—so they can buy something else they want. You are respecting their decision. It might be as easy as buying garbage cans for them to use. Remember, if they come up with the idea, then they are more likely to follow through with the organization. If you tell them how to do something, and it doesn't make sense for their personality, they either won't do it or won't do it for very long.

<u>Refrigerator Food Hoarder</u>: One of the hardest things for me to deal with is Mom's refrigerator. Part of the problem is that her eyes are failing so she cannot see into the back of the refrigerator. She cannot see into the vegetable bins so sometimes she forgets the fruits and vegetables are down there. Plus, she doesn't cook as much as she used to, but she still tends to buy more than she can use up before it spoils. Now when she needs a potato or an onion she just tells me and I just bring one to her from my home.

If your hoarder has food that spoils in the refrigerator, ask permission to remove spoiled food. Then when you leave their home, take the bag of food that is spoiled with you.

You notice that the catsup expired four years ago. (You probably have expired food in your refrigerator, too.) Ask your loved one if they think it's wise to make sure that they don't get food poisoning. Explain that the catsup is four years old and it can make them sick. Ask them that so you don't get sick from eating this really expired catsup, do I have your permission to remove it. If they say yes, put the catsup in your bag to go out when you leave. If they say balk, then on the next visit, when they haven't reached their time tolerance level yet, tell them the same thing and ask if you can remove the expired catsup so that it doesn't make them sick.

Thank them for all that <u>they</u> got accomplished today.   Once they finish the project, praise them.

<u>Restaurant Take-Out Container Hoarding</u>: This category probably really frustrates non hoarders.   To you, the restaurant take-out container hoarder is keeping trash. For some of us hoarders, we reuse the containers because most of them do not break down in the landfills; especially Styrofoam containers.

How to help your restaurant take-out container hoarder. Ask your loved one, nicely, if, today, we can look at their restaurant take-out containers.   It's going to be hard, but don't complain or mumble underneath your breath about keeping garbage or your loved one will feel disrespected and shut down and that will be the end of the downsizing session today. Depending on how much you distress your loved one, it might also send them into a hoarding-buying frenzy.

After all of the containers have been collected, sort them according to size and type of material. You should have a pile of Styrofoam containers, in various sizes, as well as plastic containers.

If they have cardboard take-out containers, ask them if they think it's smart to do things so we won't get food poisoning. (We always want to phrase questions so they are answering yes.) Point to the cardboard containers and explain, nicely, that they are manufactured as a one-time use container. To reuse them, could cause a person to get sick. Ask them if they want to stay healthy. Ask them if you can remove the cardboard containers from the pile. If yes, then put them in the pile that will go with you when you leave. If the containers are dirty, they need to be thrown out. If they have been washed, they can be recycled. If your loved one balks, keep calm. Ask them if it's okay if you put them in a (marked and dated) box and put it in the garage.

Look on the bottom of the plastic containers for the recycling code. Separate the containers into two piles: recyclable and non-recyclable.

Ask them that since they have plastic containers that cannot be recycled, is it okay if you take the containers that can be recycled and recycle them. If they say yes, then put them in the bag or box to go. If they balk, then ask if it would be okay if you put them in a (marked and dated) box and put it in the garage for now.

Ask them if there is a reason they are keeping the remaining containers (which are the non-recyclable plastic containers and the Styrofoam containers). Listen to their answer. If they won't budge, then ask them if you can put them in a (marked and dated) box and put the box in the garage.

Another tactic, which might or might not work, is to ask your loved one if you could remove the containers if they would start taking their own to-go containers from home to restaurants. Most restaurants are glad that you do this because it saves them in the cost of the containers. It should not be a surprise that I try to take to-go containers from home with me. These containers have tight sealing lids; the restaurant to-go containers do not.

I'm not sure if this would help your loved one or not. In my bedroom I have three bags of to-go containers and other containers that I'm willing to part with. (Lunch meat came in some of them.) Once a month I attend a potluck where people can take home dishes if they like them. I take a bunch of these containers to the potluck and donate them to the potluck. It makes me feel a little better that I can do something with the containers.

When you are done, thank your loved one for what <u>they</u> got accomplished today. When you leave, take all of the containers with you that will be donated, recycled, or thrown in the trash. Once you are done with the project, praise them.

<u>Rubber Band Hoarding</u>: If you wonder why I'm including such a minor category, it's because people do hoard rubber bands and if we can get your hoarder to conquer one area of hoarding, even minor, it will give them confidence that they can handle more emotionally difficult downsizing.

This category probably is another category that really frustrates non hoarders. To you, you only need a few rubber bands in your office. Often fresh vegetables come wrapped with a rubber band.

How to help your rubber band hoarder: Ask your loved one, nicely, if, today, we can look at their rubber bands. It's going to be hard, but don't complain or mumble underneath your breath about keeping hundreds of rubber bands. If your loved one hears you, they will feel disrespected and shut down and that will be the end of the downsizing session today. Depending on how much you distress your loved one, it might also send them into a hoarding-buying frenzy.

As you are sorting the rubber bands according to size, stretch all of the rubber bands and put all of the dry-rotted rubber bands that break in one pile. Ask your loved one if you can remove all of the broken rubber bands. Put them in your box to go.

Ask them, nicely, if there is a reason they are keeping so many rubber bands. Listen to their answer. If they balk, ask them if you can put them in a (marked and dated) box and put the box in the garage.

Ask your loved one which size of rubber bands they use the most. Ask them if a dozen is enough to keep on hand. Honor their wishes. Ask them if you can donate some of the rubber bands. Put all of the rubber bands that they will let go in the box to go to donate. If they balk, put them in a (marked and dated) box and put in the garage.

When you are done, thank your loved one for what <u>they</u> got accomplished today. When you leave, take all of the rubber bands with you that will be donated, recycled, or thrown in the trash. When they have finished this project, praise your loved one.

<u>Salt & Pepper Packet and Sugar Packet Hoarder</u>: If your loved one has saved salt & pepper packets, sugar packets, and similar types of packets, from restaurants, ask them if we can look at them today. Gather them all up and sort by the item: salt, pepper, sugar, and whatever other packet they have.

Ask them if they enjoy helping other people out. If they say yes, ask them if they would like to help others out by donating the packets. If yes, put them in a bag to go. If they balk, ask them if they would rather donate the packets or spend the time breaking them open and putting them into the shakers. They may or may not agree to let the salt and pepper be donated and keep the sugar. Whatever they agree to keep, get out the container, and start ripping the packets and adding them to the container; i.e. sugar packets are poured into the sugar container.

When you are done, thank your loved one for what <u>they</u> got accomplished today. When you leave, take all packets with you that they offered to donate.   Once they finish the project, praise them.

<u>Shoe Hoarding</u>: Most likely their bedroom is a mess with clothes, shoes, and other stuff all over the place. If you know that they enjoy buying shoes, instead of tackling their room, you might ask them if it's okay if, today, we organize just their shoes.

Don't say anything about the mess in their room or that they only can wear one pair of shoes at a time. It's about them and not about you.

Pull out all of their shoes, boots, athletic shoes (sneakers), and slippers. If you only can find one shoe of a pair, ask them nicely if they might know where the other shoe is. So now you have stacks of shoes. (I'm not a shoe hoarder so, I'm like you and don't understand why they need dozens of shoes.)

While you are doing this, ask nicely, what thrift store charities that they enjoy that are nearby. If you know that the thrift store that they mentioned doesn't take clothing, keep asking until in your mind you have one that will take the items.

Ask them if any of the shoes they just don't like. If they mention one or more, pull them out of the stack and start a separate pile. Ask them if any of the shoes hurt their feet; that they just don't fit right. Add those shoes to the separate pile.

Now you really have to be careful how you word things or you are going to increase your loved one's stress level and today's sorting is basically done.

Say your loved one likes to garden. You see several pair of worn sneakers or other shoes. Pull them out of the pile. Nicely ask them if all of these are their gardening shoes. If they say no, put them to the edge of the pile to be sorted. If they say yes, ask them if any of the shoes leak. If yes, put them in a new pile. Ask them if any of the gardening shoes hurt their feet. Again, put them in the new pile. Say you still have more than one pair of gardening shoes/boots left. Ask them which pair of gardening shoes do they like the best. Put those shoes in a new pile. If they balk and say they wear two pair, then tell them okay and keep two pair out in the new keep pile.

By now their time tolerance is probably getting near their limit. Your emphasis is now on the pile with the worn shoes and the shoes they don't like or don't fit well anymore.

For the shoes that they don't like or that don't fit well anymore. Remind them of all the good that their favorite charity does. Since you don't like these shoes and these shoes really hurt your feet, is it okay for me to donate to their charity. If they say yes, box or bag up those shoes and put by the door to go with you. If they say they aren't ready to get rid of those shoes yet, keep calm. Ask them if it's okay if you box them and put them in the garage. If yes, then next time, when their time tolerance is low, you can ask again and they should be more receptive to donating them.

Now to the gardening shoes that are so beat up that they cannot be donated. I would point to the gardening shoes that they are keeping and nicely remind them that they really like those gardening shoes. Ask them if it is okay to pull the shoe strings out of these other gardening shoes. They should say okay. (It's always less stressful if at least part of an item can be salvaged.) Remind them that these shoes leak or are worn down so that they might cause knee or back pain when they wear them. Ask them if it's okay if you take them with you. If they say that it's okay, put them by your pile to go. These shoes can be thrown out; whereas, the other shoes can be donated.

Their time tolerance is gone by now. Ask them if it's okay for you to box the rest of the shoes up for now; that you are done for today and you are proud of them for what <u>they</u> got accomplished today.

The next visit. Back to the bedroom or other room where your loved one keeps their shoes. Ask them if they have thought about the remaining shoes and there are more that they don't like or they just don't fit right. It's doubtful, but they actually might surprise you and offer to get rid of more shoes.

Today you are going to use a different angle. For each type of shoe you are going to ask which their favorite is: shoes, sneakers, sandals, and slippers. Pull them out to keep. If they really like others, then pull them out too.

Then sort the remaining shoes by category. Ask them if there are any shoes that don't go with any of their outfits. Pull them and put them in a new pile.

Ask them if there are any shoes that they haven't worn in over a year. Pull them out and add to the new pile. (This might start to cause them some anxiety.)

If they have several shoes of the same color, ask them which one they like the best and want to keep. Pull that out in the save pile and the others in the new pile.

You now have a stack of shoes, boots, sneakers, and slipper pile. Point to the black shoes that they kept out. Remind them that they wanted to keep, pointing, to those black shoes. Ask them if it's okay if you donate the other black shoes to their favorite charity. Go through that entire pile. At this point, they might really be getting stressed out and don't want to get rid of any of that pile. You need to immediately stop and praise them for what <u>they</u> got done today. Tell them that you are not going to do anything with these shoes; you are just going to put them in the box. Ask them if it's okay if you put just this (marked) box in the garage.

Next trip, when their stress time tolerance is low, you can ask about the shoes in the garage. You can remind them that last time they were about to donate that box of shoes to their favorite charity. Ask them if it's okay if you do that. They might pull one or even all of the shoes out of the box now wanting to keep them. Keep calm. Don't yell at them out of frustration. This is about them and has nothing to do with you.

They need to decide what zone their shoes will be kept in.

If you've downsized any, it's better than it was before you started. You have to be grateful for even the baby steps.

Thank them for all that <u>they</u> accomplished today. Once the project is done, praise them for completing the project.

<u>Used Napkins and Paper Towels</u>: This one is going to try your patience. You do not understand why your loved one is saving trash. This also includes new napkins that they have brought home from restaurants.

In a nonjudgmental voice, ask them if there is a reason why they are keeping used napkins and paper towels. Listen to, and respect, their answer.

Yes, I am a used napkin and paper towel hoarder. And, yes, I do have a zone near the kitchen. Probably surprisingly to you, there are times that I've almost run out of them.

There are two basic reasons I save them. When restaurants give us paper napkins, and even though we don't use them, they are supposed to throw them out which is wasting the resources that God has given us. Some restaurants put small napkins underneath the beverage glass. They are perfectly clean; they just need to be dried out. Besides being a hoarder, I'm cheap—or thrifty as I like to say. If I can avoid having a plumber come to the house I will do it. If you are wondering what that has to do with hoarding junk, keep reading. Certain foods are cooked in oil, butter, or are greasy by nature. Instead of just dumping that grease down the drain, when the dishes are washed, thus increasing the chance of it eventually clogging up and having to pay a plumber over $100 to come into my house to fix it, I'm proactive. I use the used paper towels and napkins to wipe off greasy utensils and use them to wipe out pans prior to washing. If we are eating wings, we will use the unused paper napkins brought home from restaurants. (I don't purposefully take excess paper napkins from the restaurant's paper napkin holders with the sole intent to bring home. I'm sure that some hoarders might.)

This might surprise you, but for me, this hoarding item is nonnegotiable. If I got rid of the used napkins, then it would be wasteful to use clean paper towels to do the same thing because I will continue to wipe out greasy pans before washing.

I have a zone that the used napkins and paper towels go into, which is right at the edge of the kitchen. It's a nice-looking wood file cabinet that been used for different functions throughout the years. It has two drawers in it. The top 3.5" deep drawer is used for the used napkins and paper towels. The bottom drawer, which is deep enough for file folders, is where I stash my bags; i.e. bread bags, and various sized bags from different items. Store bags are kept in a different zone.

If your loved one keeps really dirty used napkins and paper towels, ask them if they are willing to do something that would help keep roaches out of their house. They should say yes. In a nice tone of voice, ask them if it is okay <u>just</u> to remove the really dirty used napkins and paper towels so that they don't attract roaches. Put them in a bag to take home with you, today, (so that they won't possibly pull them out of their trash and hide them where they think you won't find them).

Same thing with moldy used napkins and paper towels. Instead of saying roaches, you want to phrase your question about them doing something that would help them to not get sick. Make sure that the question is worded so that the answer is yes.

What works for me might not seem logical to your loved one. Ask your loved one if <u>they</u> have any ideas how <u>they</u> would like to organize their used napkins and paper towels. Listen to their answer. Remember, if you suggest or make them do something that is not logical to them, they won't do it for long—if at all.

If your loved one is unclear of what to do, you might ask them if you can offer some suggestions. One suggestion might be to use one of the cloth bags that they still probably have too many of.   You could use a nonexpendable or one that expands at the bottom. Ask them that if you put a hook right inside of their pantry door, and hook the bag to it, would they be willing to keep all of their used napkins and paper towels in it. If they say yes, great. You might want to put up several hooks; one could be for the used napkins and paper towels. Another hook could be used to hang aprons. Again, you want to empower your loved one so that they will feel good that you didn't criticize them.   We, meaning hoarders, know that you think most/all of our stuff is junk. But, if you treat <u>us</u> and our stuff respectful, we feel respected and will be more receptive to work on other areas and keep our zones cleaner.

Thank them for all that <u>they</u> accomplished today. When they have completed this project, praise them.

<center>~~~</center>

In summary. By now you have worked <u>with</u> your loved one on downsizing specific items down to levels that their anxiety level can handle. If you were too forceful, that will soon become quite evident as they will start hoarding those items, again, or will go on a hoarding-buying binge to calm their nerves.

The next section will discuss working on zones, or areas where you most likely wanted to start with first. But if you have read the book and have implemented the suggestions written in this book, then you should understand why we started with specific items first. Now they should be more receptive to working in zones, which are specific areas within their home, garage, and yard.

Part III

How to help your hoarder: zones

How to Help your Hoarder: Zones

If you have not read Part I or Part II yet, please go back and read them in order so that you can help your hoarder in the quickest most efficient manner. If you just jump in without understanding how hoarders, of which I am one, thinks, you might do or say something that sends your loved one off the edge, alienate you from them, and your tone, words and/or actions could cause them so much anxiety that they go on a hoarding buying spree.

If you are really serious and sincere about helping your hoarder, then read Part I followed by Part II and then come back to Part III where I talk about zones.

> Before working on zones, you need to work on four; preferably more specific types of hoarding items. Why? Because zones are <u>WAY</u> more anxiety producing than specific items.

By now you hopefully understand your loved one, who just happens to be a hoarder. You'll never understand hoarding; you don't have to. Like I said previously, I do not understand how a car runs, but I still drive one.

You understand that it's not about you; it's about your loved one and how you can help them get control of their life—if you do it in a way that makes them feel respected and listened to.

In Part II you worked with your loved one, in a dignified way, to reduce some of their hoarding by putting your energy into specific types of hoarding and you helped your loved one work through and reduce some of their hoarding clutter.

Now you are going to work on specific zones. In the most simplistic of terms, a zone is a specific area. It could be your loved one's trunk or the inside of their vehicle, or their kitchen counter, bathroom counter, bathroom, bedroom, garage, or other cluttered zone.

> You don't start with a huge zone like their living room or you will probably fail miserably and increase your loved one's anxiety, which might trigger a hoarding shopping spree.

I will be your coach and, together, we will work to try to empower your loved one to tackle zones, one zone at a time, in their home, garage, yard, and vehicle.

If you are ready to help your loved one further, please go to the next page.

Easy Zones

Since you and your loved one have been working, together, on specific items that they have been hoarding, you might see less clutter when you enter their home, garage, vehicle, and/or yard.

Now we are stepping it up a little as you and your loved one tackle zones.

By empowering your loved one, who just happens to be a hoarder, they hopefully should be feeling good about the changes that they have made--if you have handled downsizing specific items correctly.

After you feel that you have worked on enough specific areas, ask them if it would be okay to look at zones. When they look confused and ask you what a zone is, you tell them that it is a specific area that <u>they</u> pick to work on. Reassure your loved one that they will pick the zone; they are in total control of the zone. Ask them if it would be okay for them to pick an easy zone. If they are ready, they will say yes.

<h1 style="text-align:center">Easy Zones</h1>

- ➢ Vehicle trunk
- ➢ Dresser top
- ➢ Bathroom counter
- ➢ Purse, backpack, or briefcase
- ➢ Other

Other is any other zone that they pick.

You ask your loved one if they would like to start with their vehicle trunk, their dresser top, their bathroom counter, their purse (or backpack or briefcase), or if they would rather start with something else. If your loved one doesn't own a vehicle, you wouldn't mention their trunk as an easy zone. Whatever zone they pick, is the zone you will work on first.

We're going to go through each scenario. If they picked something else, the same principles apply to the zone they suggest and you just let them rearrange the picking of their easy zones to the order they wish to complete them.

<u>Vehicle trunk</u>: Ask them if they would be more comfortable if we empty everything in the trunk (minus the spare tire, tire rod, and jack) into

boxes and bring them inside. If they agree, put everything into several boxes and cart them inside without mumbling or complaining. If they reply that they would rather work outside, ask them if they would like you to bring a chair outside for them to sit in.

As you are emptying the trunk into boxes, try to put similar items in to the same box as you are filling up the boxes.

Tackle one box at a time. Have several marked boxes or bags:

<u>Take</u> (In this box goes trash and other items which are not good enough to donate. You do not call the items trash.)

<u>Donate</u> (Items in which your loved one has agreed to donate to a charity thrift store or other place.)

<u>Recycle</u> (Items that can be recycled such as plastic bottles, glass, cans, paper, etc.)

<u>Keep—trunk</u> (Loved one wants to keep the item in their trunk.)

<u>Keep-other</u> (Loved one wants to keep the item, but not in their trunk.)

Go through one box at a time. Ask if it's okay to remove items such as food wrappers, used straws, and obvious trash. Do not call the items trash. Show them the items and if they agree, put them in the trash box which you call the other box. If there are empty bottles, cans, or other items that can be recycled, ask your loved one if you can recycle these items. Put them in the recycle box. If there are water bottles with water still in them, put them in the recycle box and then later empty the water bottles. Check the water bottle tops to see if they can be recycled. If they can, unscrew the bottle tops and when you recycle the bottles, the recyclable top should be loose and not attached to the plastic bottle. Put them in the recycle box.

If you find maps in their trunk, and they still use maps, ask them if they would like them put inside of their vehicle where they are more easily accessible. If they have duplicate maps, ask them which map they would prefer to keep in their vehicle. Ask if they would rather donate or recycle the duplicate maps (if the map is good enough to donate). Ask them where they want to store the duplicate maps they are keeping.

> The objective remains the same—we are trying to find a place to put everything—that makes sense to your loved one.

If there are outdated newspapers or magazines in the boxes, ask if they can be recycled (or donated). If they want to keep them, then pull out of all of the newspapers and magazines from the boxes and put those with the other newspapers and magazines you have previously gone through that are already neatly stacked in marked boxes.

If there are papers, ask if each paper can be recycled or shredded (if it has any personal information on it). Put in the appropriate box. Papers that they want to keep, ask where they wish to put them.

By the time you finish going through the boxes, their time tolerance should be done. If there are still papers or other items you need to go through, ask your loved one if they want to finish the box or if they want to do it on your next visit. If they want to wait, mark another box with the date to work on next visit. Then put the items that they want back in their trunk in a box or another storage container.

Thank them for all that <u>they</u> accomplished today and take the boxes with you to donate, recycle, and/or throw away. When they have finished with this zone, congratulate them on cleaning an entire zone.

<u>Dresser top</u>: Ask your loved one if you can put everything on their bed. (If their bed is not made, cover the sheets with a bedspread or blanket.) Ask them if they would rather sit on the edge of the bed or in a chair (if a chair can fit in their bedroom with all of their other clutter). As you are putting everything on their bed, try to sort the items into piles of like things such as change in one pile.

If there is money as a pile, ask them where they want to put their money. If in a purse, ask them which purse it is, and ask them if they would like to put their money in their purse. If they don't want to do anything with the money, ask them if you can get a bowl and put the money in there. If yes, put the money in the bowl and ask them if they want the bowl put back on their dresser.

Pick up and ask if it's okay to remove items such as food wrappers and drink cans and water bottles. Do not call the items trash. Show them the items and if they agree, put wrappers in the trash box. If there are empty bottles, cans, or other items that can be recycled, ask your loved one if you can recycle these items. Put them in the recycle box. If there are water bottles with water still in them, put them in the recycle box and then later empty the water bottles. Check the water bottle tops to see if they can be recycled. If they can, unscrew the bottle tops and put them in the recycle box separately.

For everything else on their bed, go through each thing and ask your loved one where they want to put the item. Items that can be put away, put away.

Ask your loved one if they would like you to dust the top of their dresser.

Thank them for all that <u>they</u> accomplished today and take the boxes with you to donate, recycle, and/or throw away. When they have finished with this zone, congratulate them on cleaning an entire zone.

<u>Bathroom counter</u>: The bathroom counter was one of the easiest zones for me to work on and to maintain for weeks now.

Ask your loved one if they would rather work on the bathroom counter zone in the bathroom or bring everything to the bed. (If they choose their bed, cover their sheets with a bedspread or blanket.) Work on groups of the same item at the same time.

Ask your loved one if there are any items that they don't use anymore. If they point out one or more things, ask them if you can put them in the box (to recycle, donate, or throw out later). Then go through each item and have them decide where to put it.

What works for you probably may or may not work for your loved one. In order for them to keep a zone clean, it has to make sense to them. That's why you keep asking them where <u>they</u> would like to put an item.

Clean their bathroom countertop and their sink and mirror. Ask them if there is anything that would make them happy to attach to the corner of their mirror. Ask them if there is something small that would make them happy if it was put on their counter. Ask them if they would like to put a towel, nearby, so they could easily wipe off the countertop, faucet, and sink. If they do, ask them what small towel or cloth and where would they like to keep it.

What I did was to put and keep my toothpaste in one of the sink drawers where it immediately goes back into after I'm done with it. The bottle of mouthwash, when I'm not using it, goes right inside of the bottom cupboard doors. I keep a small towel draped over the bottom cabinet door and after I'm done washing my hands or brushing my teeth, I wipe off the faucet and counter top. Then on the counter, in the corners, I put something that makes me happy. I also put something on the corner of my mirrors that makes me happy. So, now, I love my bathroom counter top; it makes me feel good and I <u>want</u> to keep it clutter free!

If your loved one still wishes to keep one or more items on their bathroom counter, honor their request.

Thank them for all that <u>they</u> accomplished today and take the boxes with you to donate, recycle, and/or throw away. When they have finished with this zone, congratulate them on cleaning an entire zone.

<u>Purse, backpack, or briefcase</u>: I'm going to mention cleaning out their purse; however, the same concepts work if they use a backpack or briefcase.

Ask your loved one where they would like to empty out their purse (or backpack or briefcase). Ask if you can remove (don't say throw out) wrappers, drink bottles, or empty cans. Since this is a pretty small zone, you can use one box or bag and put everything in it and sort it out into donate, recycle, or trash when you get home.

If your loved one has more than two pens in their purse, ask them which two pens and one pencil (if there are pencils in their purse) they would like to remain in their purse. Have a piece of scratch paper to test the pens to make sure that they still work. Ask if you can put the remaining pens and pencils in with their other pens and pencils.

If they have more than one Chap Stick type item, lipstick, or other similar item, ask them which Chap Stick type item (or lipstick or other similar item) they want to keep in their purse. Ask if you can put the others with the other items (that you have already sorted, with them, previously).

> Go through each remaining item and ask them where they want it put because if you ask them if they want it to stay in their purse, they will say yes to almost everything.

Thank them for all that _they_ accomplished today and take the boxes with you to donate, recycle, and/or throw away. When they have finished with this zone, congratulate them on cleaning an entire zone.

~~~

How are they doing? Have they backslid? If they have, don't be judgmental. It could be that they tried something and when they did, it didn't make sense. Just readjust and ask them what else they think _they_ would be willing to try that would help. (Their backsliding could be in a specific area such as paper building up, again or in zones such as keeping their trunk neat.)
~~~

Remember, it took them years to accumulate all of their clutter. It may take a couple of tries for them to adapt to a new way of living with their stuff in a more organized manner. Be supportive and not critical.

Always thank your loved one for what <u>they</u> accomplished, today. Praise them after they complete each zone.

Moderate Zones

Before moving to moderate zones, casually look around and see if you need to work on maintenance first. Maintenance is when your loved one has gotten a little lax with prior specific hoarding items or prior zones. Say you start to see more restaurant take-out containers lying around. Don't shame them. Don't make negative comments about their clutter accumulation in items and/or zones that were previously worked on. Nicely, and in a nonjudgmental tone, ask your loved what they would suggest to make it easier with their, in this case, restaurant take-out containers, items. (Don't call it trash, or clutter, or other insulting names.) Really listen. It might just be that the location of the zone for the restaurant take-out containers might just need to be moved. They might be more receptive for them to be recycled. Nicely ask them if it would be okay to recycle the extra take-out containers. If so, put them in the recycle box to go when you leave for the day.

You should be able to judge whether or not your loved one is able and willing to tackle moderate zones. When you visit your loved one, who just happens to be a hoarder, you don't <u>always</u> have to work on their clutter. You can just visit and enjoy each other's company.

The best way to know is to ask your loved one if they would like to hear what the moderate zones are and if they would like to pick one. This makes your loved one feel empowered and feel like that they are in control which reduces their anxiety level.

<u>Moderate Zones</u>
- ➢ Vehicle: inside
- ➢ Kitchen counter
- ➢ Coat closet
- ➢ Laundry room or area
- ➢ Other

Other is any other zone that they pick.

Ask your loved one if they would like to start with the inside of their vehicle, their kitchen counter, their laundry room (or laundry area; whichever they have), or something else. If your loved one doesn't own a vehicle or a washer and dryer, you wouldn't mention that as a moderate zone. Whatever zone they pick, is the zone you will work on first.

We're going to go through each scenario. If they picked something else, the same principles apply to the zone they suggest.

<u>Vehicle: inside</u>: Ask them if they would be more comfortable if we empty everything that's in their car into boxes and bring them inside. If they agree, put everything into several boxes and cart them inside without mumbling or complaining. If they reply that they would rather work outside, ask them if they would like you to bring a chair outside for them to sit in.

To save time, later, as you are emptying out their vehicle, try to put similar items in the same box.

Tackle one box at a time. Depending on how much stuff they have in their vehicle will determine how many sort boxes you will need. If you need several boxes, you can label them as:

<u>Take</u> (You will take the item, which is garbage or the item isn't good enough to recycle or donate.)

<u>Donate</u> (You will take the item when you leave for the day and donate it.)

150

<u>Recycle</u> (You will take the item when you leave for the day and recycle it.)

<u>Keep—vehicle</u> (Loved one wants to keep the item in their vehicle.)

<u>Keep-other</u> (Loved one wants to keep the item, but not in their vehicle.)

Go through one box at a time. Ask if it's okay to remove items such as food wrappers, used straws, and obvious trash. Do not call the items trash. Show them the items and if they agree, put them in the remove (trash) box. If there are empty bottles, cans, or other items that can be recycled, ask your loved one if you can recycle these items. Put them in the recycle box. If there are water bottles with water still in them, put them in the recycle box and then later empty the water bottles. Check the water bottle tops to see if they can be recycled. If they can, unscrew the bottle tops and put them in the recycle box separately.

If they have maps, and they still use maps, ask them if they would like them put inside of their vehicle where they are more easily accessible. If they have duplicate maps, ask them which map they would prefer to keep in their vehicle.

Ask if they would rather donate or recycle the map (if the map is good enough to donate). If they decide to keep duplicate maps, ask where they would like to store them.

If there are outdated newspapers or magazines in the boxes, ask if they can be recycled (or donated). If they want to keep them, then pull out of all of the newspapers and magazines and put them with the other newspapers and magazines that were previously sorted and boxed.

If there are papers, ask if each paper can be recycled or shredded (if it has any personal information on it). Put in the appropriate box. Papers that they want to keep, ask where they want to put them.

If there is clothing, ask if they want it in their laundry basket to be washed. Some clothing may go back in their vehicle. I generally have a ball cap in the car in case the sun is low and hitting me in the face. It's okay for them to have some items in their vehicle.

There might be one or more bags of purchases that just haven't made it into their house yet. Go through each bag and ask them where they want each item to go.

By the time you finish going through the boxes, their time tolerance should be done. If there's still papers or other items you need to go through, ask your loved one if they want to finish the box or if they want to do it on your next visit. If they want to wait, mark another bag or box with the date to work on next visit. Then put the items that they want back in their vehicle.

Thank your loved one for all that <u>they</u> accomplished today. Take the boxes with you to donate, recycle, and/or throw away. Praise your loved one once they finish this zone.

<u>Kitchen counter</u>: Ask your loved one if they would like to work on their kitchen counter today.   Empower your loved one by asking them if they want their toaster and coffee pot, (if they own them), to stay on the counter. Most people do have these items on their counter.

There may be a few to a lot of dirty dishes all over their counter. Ask them for their opinion. In a nonjudgmental voice, ask them if there is a reason for the dirty dishes. Say if and not why because it sounds less judgmental. It could be as simple that they are out of dish detergent or their dishwasher is broken. If that is not the reason for the dirty dishes, ask them, nicely and in a nice tone, how they would like to tackle the dirty dishes. If they don't know, then you can offer suggestions. One suggestion, which you might not like, is for you to manually wash the dishes without complaining or mumbling under your breath. You can do the dishes while talking about other pleasant subjects besides the dirty dishes or their clutter. Or, if they have a working dishwasher, you can empty their dishwasher and load and start the dishwasher with the first load.

If there is change, magazines, or newspapers on the counter, ask if you can put it with the other change, magazines, or newspapers.

If there is unopened or opened mail, ask them if it would be okay if, together, you could go through the mail. For junk mail (don't call it junk mail) and pleas for donations, ask them if you can take that mail home to shred and recycle the paper. Set all bills aside, momentarily, until the mail has been sorted. After you have gone through all of their mail, ask them if they would like you to help them get these bills done and out of the way so that they don't have to worry about them anymore.

For the remaining items on their counter, ask them what they would like to do with each item and honor their requests. By now, you are most likely past their time tolerance.

If it this zone takes more than one day to complete, thank them for what <u>they</u> accomplished, today. Praise them when they have completed this zone.

<u>Coat closet</u>: Ask your loved one if they would like to work on their coat closet today. Ask them how they would like to tackle the project; whether they would like to start with the hanging items, the top shelf (if any) or their items on the floor.

<u>Top shelf</u>: You probably need a step stool or step ladder to safely pull everything off of the shelf. Ask your loved one if there is anything that they don't like or use anymore that they want to donate or recycle it. If so, pull that aside. Go through each item and have them decide what they would like to do with it. Ask them their opinion on how to organize the top shelf better. (It might be to get some small

plastic containers with tops to keep some of the items organized better.) At this point your loved one's time tolerance should be near. Ask them if they wish to continue or wait until your next visit. If they are done for the day, praise them for all <u>they</u> accomplished, today.

<u>Hanging items</u>: Ask your loved one how they want to tackle these items.   Once suggestion is to haul everything to one of the made-up beds and go through each item.

You might want to group certain items such as jackets in one group, snow pants in another group, rain gear in one group, and winter coats in another group. For each group ask them if there are any that they don't like, they don't fit, or they don't want anymore. Ask if you can donate the items and put them in bags or boxes. If they have two or more items that are very similar, ask them which one they would like to keep and set that in the save pile. Ask them if it would be okay to donate the rest. Honor their decision—either way.   If they have miscellaneous items that really don't belong in the coat closet such as blouses or shirts, ask if there is a reason they are in the coat closet. You can ask if it is okay to move them to their bedroom closet.

Once they have made a decision on all of the items, hang up the clothing they are going to save. Ask your loved one, first, the order they want their hanging clothes; meaning do they want the coats on the left or the right. If they still have quite a few items hanging, ask them if they would like a hanging rack to be attached to the inside of the closet door where they can hang up a few jackets, scarfs, and hats. If they want it, ask them if they would like to go be with you when you to pick one out on your next visit or if they would like you to pick something out. (Choices are plastic, wood, or metal hooks or knobs that are single or several attached to the base. If it's plastic, there might be several colors to choose from.)

At this point your loved one's time tolerance should be past.   If they are done for the day, praise them for all <u>they</u> accomplished today. Congratulate them for finishing part of a moderate project.

   <u>Coat closet floor</u>: Ask them if it's okay to pull everything out from the floor of the closet. (You might be shocked how much stuff they have crammed into their closet.) Don't be judgmental or complain or your loved one will shut down and that will be the end of their downsizing.

Ask your loved one if there is anything that they don't like or use anymore that they want to donate or recycle. If so, pull that aside. Go through each item and have them decide what they would like to do with it. Ask them their opinion on how to organize the area better. (It might be to get some small plastic containers with tops to keep some of the items organized better.)

Thank your loved one for all that <u>they</u> accomplished today. Take the boxes with you to donate, recycle, and/or throw away. Praise your loved one once they finish this zone.

<u>Laundry room or area</u>: Ask your loved one if they would like to work on their laundry area today. Ask them how they would like to tackle the project; whether they would like to start with the shelfs or cabinets, the items on the floor, or the items piled on the washer and dryer.

<u>Shelves or cabinets</u>: Start with the highest shelf or cabinet shelf. You might need a step stool or step ladder to reach the top shelf. There might be items on the shelves that are not related to laundry at all. Do not be critical or your loved one will shut down and that will be the end of downsizing for the day. Depending

on how crammed the shelves or cabinets are, you probably won't get to the items on the floor or piled on the washer and dryer today.

Ask your loved one if there is anything that they don't like or use anymore that they want to donate or recycle it. (Some of the items might need to be thrown out. Don't say thrown out; instead say removed.) If so, pull that aside. Go through each item and have them decide what they would like to do with it. Ask them their opinion on how to organize the area better. (It might be to get some containers with tops to keep some of the items organized better.) Most likely their time tolerance has passed. Ask if they want to continue or to stop and continue on your next visit. Thank them for what <u>they</u> have accomplished, today. When you leave for the day take all of the items to recycle, donate, or throw away. Congratulate them for finishing part of a moderate project.

<u>Items on the floor</u>: There might be anything on the floor that is not related to laundry at all. Do not be critical or your loved one will shut down and that will be the end of downsizing for the day. Depending on how crammed the floor is, you might not even get to the items piled on the washer and dryer today.

Ask your loved one if there is anything that they don't like or use anymore that they want to donate or recycle it. (Some of the items might need to be thrown out. Don't say thrown out; instead say removed.) If so, pull that aside. Go through each item and have them decide what they would like to do with it. Ask them their opinion on how to organize the area better. (It might be to get some containers with tops to keep some of the items organized better.) Most likely their time tolerance has passed. Ask if they want to continue and work on the items on the washer and dryer or to stop and continue on your next visit. Thank them for what <u>they</u> have accomplished, today. When you leave for the day take all of the items to recycle, donate, or throw away. Congratulate them when they have finished this partial moderate zone.

<u>Washer and dryer</u>: This may be the easiest area to clean up. They may either have clean or dirty clothes piled up on them. Ask them, nicely, if there is a reason that clothes are on the washer and dryer. If there are dirty clothes, ask them if they would like to start the washer. If there are wet, clean clothes, ask them if they would like to throw them in the dryer. Congratulate them when they finish the washer and dryer zone.

Since the washer and dryer are flat surfaces, it may become a handy table to dump bags of groceries or other items that they purchased or dragged home. If it's food, ask them if it would be okay if you marked the food items with their expiration date and put them away. For other items, take each bag or item and ask what they would like to do with them. If they are past their time tolerance, ask them if they would like to finish this next time.

Thank your loved one for all that <u>they</u> accomplished today. Take the boxes with you to donate, recycle, and/or throw away.   Praise your loved one once they finish this zone.

__Moderate Plus Zones__

You should be able to judge whether or not your loved one is able and willing to tackle more zones. The best way to know is to ask them if they would like to hear what some of the next zones are and if they would like to pick one.

We don't want to call them more challenging zones or that might increase their anxiety level.

Moderate Plus Zones

- ➢ Bedroom closet
- ➢ Dining room table
- ➢ Office
- ➢ Guest room
- ➢ Other

Other is any other zone that they pick.

Ask your loved one if they would like to start with their bedroom closet, their dining room table, their office, guest room, or if they would like to work on another area. If they don't have an office and/or a guest room, you won't mention that zone. Whatever zone they pick, is the zone you will work on first.

We're going to go through each scenario. If they picked something else, the same principles apply to the zone they suggest.

<u>Bedroom closet</u>: Ask your loved one how they would like to tackle the project; whether they would like to start with the top shelf, the hanging items, or their items on the floor.

Their bedroom closet zone might take several visits to complete. Make sure you are respectful of their time tolerance.

<u>Top shelf</u>: You probably need a step stool or step ladder to safely pull everything off of the shelf. Ask your loved one if there is anything that they don't like or use anymore that they want to donate or recycle it. If so, pull that aside. Go through each item and have them decide what they would like to do with it. Ask them their opinion on how to organize the top shelf better. (It might be to get some small plastic containers with tops to keep some of the items organized better.) At this point your loved one's time tolerance should be near. Ask them if they wish to continue or wait until your next

visit. If they are done for the day, praise them for all <u>they</u> accomplished, today.

<u>Hanging items</u>: Ask your loved one how they want to tackle these items. Once suggestion is to haul everything to their made-up bed and go through each item.

Group similar items together: slacks/pants/jeans, blouses, suits, dresses, skirts. For each group ask them if there are any that they don't like, they don't fit, or they don't want anymore. Ask if you can donate the items and put them in bags or boxes. If they have two or more items that are very similar, ask them which one they would like to keep and set that in the save pile. Ask them if it would be okay to donate the others. Honor their decision—either way. If there are non-clothing items in their closet, ask them if they would like to move these items to a different zone. Respect their answer because it's okay to have anything that they want in their closet.

Once they have made a decision on all of the items, hang up the clothing they are going to save. Before doing so, ask your loved one which items they want to hang in the closet first.

> Non hoarders, too, may keep several sizes of clothes; hoping that they will eventually get back to that size.

If they are saving clothes that don't fit, right now, don't complain or mutter underneath your breath. Instead, ask them if they would like to hang the clothes that don't fit on one side of their closet. If so, hang up all of the clothes that don't fit. Then ask what type of clothing they would like to hang up next. Continue until all of the clothes are hung back up in a manner that makes sense to your loved one.

If there is not enough room for all of their hanging clothes, ask them if it would be okay for them to pull <u>just a few more</u> clothes to donate. Honor their wishes.

At this point your loved one's time tolerance should be past.   Thank your loved one for all that <u>they</u> got accomplished today.   Make sure to take all of the boxes to donate, recycle, and throw away when you leave for the day.

<u>Bedroom closet floor</u>: Ask them if it's okay to pull everything out from the floor of the closet. You might be shocked how much stuff they

have crammed into their closet. Don't be judgmental or complain or your loved one will shut down and that will be the end of their downsizing.

Ask your loved one if there is anything that they don't like or use anymore that they want to donate or recycle it. If so, pull that aside. Go through each item and have them decide what they would like to do with it. Ask them their opinion on how to organize the area better. (It might be to get some containers with tops to keep some of the items organized better.)

Once you have completed the project, praise them for all that <u>they</u> accomplished today. Congratulate them for finishing a moderate plus project.

<u>Dining room table</u>: The dining room table tends to gather clutter for both hoarders and people that aren't hoarders.

Ask your loved one if you can separate everything into like piles; i.e. mail, newspapers, magazines, notes, condiments, as well as other items.

Ask them if you can recycle the newspapers and magazines or put them with the other newspapers and other magazines.

Ask your loved one what food items and spices that are on the table they would like to be put with the other food items or spices.   Put them where your loved one asks them to go.

Before you tackle the bills, go through every other item left on the dining room table and ask your loved one where they want to be put. If the papers need to be recycled or shredded, ask them if you can take them and shred and recycle them. If so, put them in a bag or box; marking the envelopes with the word "shred".

What is remaining are bills. Ask your loved one if they would like your assistance to get their bills paid and be out of the way. Honor their wishes.

Tell your loved one that you need their opinion. Ask them what <u>we</u> can do to make it easier to keep their dining room table clean. (It might be to get a basket or an organizer to put their mail and bills in.)

Once you have completed the zone, praise them for all that <u>they</u> accomplished today. Congratulate them for finishing a moderate plus zone.

<u>Office & Guest Room</u>: Depending how much clutter has been stashed in this room, this zone may take several visits; especially if the zone has a closet in it.

> You should feel <u>honored</u> that your loved one even lets you in their office. If you think that it can't be any worse than their living room or bedroom, think again. <u>If you are feeling a little grumpy or tired today, do not start on their office, today</u>. Your reaction sets the tone for the rest of the harder zones left in their house and garage.

You might be appalled when you try to open the door to their office. In fact, there might be so much stuff crammed into their office that you have to squeeze sideways to even get into their office.

Your loved one is anxiously watching your facial expression as you try to open the door to their office. <u>You have to NOT react to every square inch to a height of up to 6 feet of boxes, bags,</u>

<u>and just clutter</u>. If you open the door, keeping your mouth shut and your face without expression, and if it's not as bad as I'm suggesting it could be, then consider that a huge blessing for the day.

If every part of their office is really cluttered, you might only get a very small area of whatever you are working on, today, sorted. Yes, if their desk is piled high, it might take you two visits just to do their desk because you have to honor their time tolerance.

If their office is really out-of-control, you do not mention that. First, you should glance around the room to see if there is a lot of one item. Say they have a lot of books strewn all over their office. To solve the problem, they need a zone for the books. It could be as simple as getting a tall bookcase. You need to ask your loved one if they think that if they buy a bookcase, if they would they use it.

Since I'm anticipating that their office probably is a total clutter disaster, work on separate zones within their office. You might have to start by filling a box, taking it to another part of the house for you and your loved one to work on. Your first zone might be just to be able to open the door.

In the office there may be a lot of new items. Since they cannot find anything in the office, if they need something, they just go out and purchase it—again. Ask them it would be okay to put everything new in a box. This is true with everything in their house.

I have friends that helped their hoarder clean her clutter and they put up shelves in her garage and put all of the new items on the shelves. Before she goes to the store, to buy an item, she checks the shelves to see if the item she needs is already on the shelf.

It might be easier, at first, to box up all of the books you see. Box up all of the magazines you see. Box up, to sort in another part of the house with your loved one, drink bottles, food wrappers, dirty dishes, and what looks like trash to you.

If there are several bags with new items in them, you might grab some bags and, together, you go through them, to decide where each item goes.

There probably is a lot of loose paper. Put them, neatly, in boxes to be sorted.

> Most likely your loved one saves scrap paper, which gets mixed up with all of the other papers. Before you go on, you need to stop, and ask your loved one what type of container or box they want to save their scrap paper in.

What I did and what works great for me is that I have one of the grocery store egg boxes and the scrap paper is put in there. When I need a piece of scrap paper, I just go to my box and grab the size paper I need. By doing this, I'm not going through the same box, and the same pieces of scrap paper over and over again. It has its own zone—a box. On the side of the box, with a magic marker I wrote scrap paper.

If your loved one saves scrap paper, you aren't going to convince them to throw the paper away. By trying to do so, you are insulting and shaming your loved one. Your loved one is going to shut down and it might send your loved one on a hoarding buying spree. Instead, work with your loved one. Someday in the future, if they are feeling less anxious, they might, on their own, reduce the amount of scrap paper they are saving. For right now, that is not the point.

> Instead, to show respect to your loved one, ask your loved one where they would like to store their scrap paper.

 Just having a box or other container for their scrap paper may significantly reduce their paper clutter. Make sure that you mark the container that <u>they</u> choose, as scrap paper.

Work each area within their office as we have discussed previously. Just accept that their office may take longer to deal with than several previous zones together.

Once your loved one has completed this zone, praise them for all that <u>they</u> accomplished today. Congratulate them for finishing a moderate plus zone!

<u>Guest room</u>: Depending how much clutter has been stashed in this room, this zone may take several visits. It's common for even non hoarders to use the guest room as their junk room where they stash things behind closed doors.

Tackle one zone of their guest room at a time. It might be the dresser, top of the bed, floor, and/or closet. Use the same suggested techniques discussed previously in this book.

Always honor your loved one's decisions. Always honor their time tolerance.

Once your loved one has completed this zone, praise them for all that <u>they</u> accomplished today. Congratulate them for finishing a moderate plus zone.

~~~

Take a deep, cleansing breath. These were some harder zones; especially sorting their office and guest room.

You and your loved one might want to take a break. These were harder zones to tackle—for your loved one and for you. You can work on maintenance with your loved one, which is areas where you might see some clutter starting to accumulate where you've already worked on the item or zone. Don't judge. Don't shame. In a nice tone, ask your loved one, to make more room for items that make them happy, if it would be okay to donate or recycle
~~~

the extra _____ that you notice. Listen to what they say. If the item is able to be donated or recycled, ask your loved one if it would be okay if they donated or recycled it. If the balk, ask them if it would be okay to donate or recycle only a few of them.

Huge Zones

You've worked with your loved one, who is a hoarder, to tackle specific items as well as some zones. Now you and your loved one can tackle any of the remaining zones which could include their living room, dining room, bedroom, hallways, porches, cellar, attic, garage, storage shed(s), storage unit(s), and/or yard.

My suggestion would work on zones which have the most trip hazard or file hazard such as their living room, kitchen, hallways, or to declutter around an outside door.

No matter if you are working on maintenance or a new zone, refer to the following list to use as your guide to increase your chances of success with your loved one. No matter which zone you work on, the same recommended concepts are the same:

1. Ask and don't tell.

2. Respect and don't shame.

3. Work within their time tolerance; the time before they start to get anxious and grumpy.

4. Ask your loved one their opinion on how to tackle their specific item or zone.

5. Really listen to your loved one.

6. Don't remove items without your loved one's permission.

7. Always word questions so the answer should be yes.

8. When you leave for the day, always take everything that is to be donated, recycled, or thrown out.

9. Always thank your loved one for what <u>they</u> got accomplished, today.

10.   It's about your loved one and never about you, so don't take it personally.

11.   Praise your loved one when they finish a zone.

12.   With your loved one's permission, put all new items in one place.

13.   If your loved one hoards something, even if you think its trash, they have an emotional attachment to it.

14.   When you clean up your loved one's clutter and take the items to put in the trash, <u>without</u> their permission, it's stealing.

15.   When you have reached or passed your loved one's time tolerance, they will start to balk at recycling or donating items. Stop. Nicely put everything away that you were working on, and thank your loved one for what <u>they</u> accomplished today.

On bigger zones, always break down the zone into mini zones; areas within the zone that you think you can work on within their time tolerance.

For instance, say your loved one wants to work on their living room. You might start with the area immediately around their chair or couch that they sit in the most. The end table or coffee table could be piled with clutter. That would probably be the most logical mini zone to start at.

If you were working on an enclosed porch, the project might be, today, just to clear a space so that your loved one could get out of the door in case of a fire or other emergency. Items could be boxed and worked in another area, where your loved one makes decisions on what to do with each item.

In the garage, it could be to clear a path to get into the house such as steps, if any, leading into the house. Box up the items on the steps and work on that box inside of the house and put where your loved one wants them.

Most likely your loved one parks in their driveway or on the road because they cannot get their vehicle into their garage.

It took me over three years before I could get my car into the garage after moving to my present residence. The sides are still stacked with boxes, however, the stacks don't go to the ceiling anymore.

What you need to really understand and respect is your loved one's time tolerance. I'd push myself past my time tolerance and get so burned out that I couldn't work on downsizing again for days or weeks. So I was working against myself instead of working, smartly, within my own time tolerance.

By now, you've made noticeable improvements with your loved one's clutter. Hopefully, this experience has brought you closer to your loved one, which is a bonus!

Thank you for treating your loved one with dignity and respect and honoring their time tolerance.

Sue